PALEO WITH A PURPOSE

Eliminate the myths once and for all.
Food; what works, what doesn't and
what you can start doing today.

JOSH BUNCH

Real Eating For Real Life
For Entertainment Purposes Only!

ISBN: 1523437286
ISBN 13: 9781523437283

TABLE OF CONTENTS

PROLOGUE

That ringtone still echoes in my ear.

My stomach dances that seaward shift and I can feel the cotton shirt I was folding.

"Josh, your uncle's on the phone," a co-worker said.

My uncle had never called me in my entire life. Much less at work; a job I wasn't entirely sure he knew I had. Immediately I thought the worst, what I got may have been just the blessing I needed, but it still didn't come easy. Blessings rarely do.

"Your dad had a stroke," uncle Larry said. "He's alive and in the hospital. Here's the address … sorry,"

Click.

That's about the gist of it. A less than one minute life changing phone call. So much for family unity, huh? Maybe that's why I value friendships so much.

Until then my dad and I didn't have a relationship. But he was still my dad, so I rushed to meet him. He was as vulnerable as a newborn. Tubes, I.V.'s and doctors surrounded him like a gate. For the first time in a long time, possibly ever, I wanted my dad. I needed to know he was ok.

My father (48-years-old at the time) was the picture of what not to do. From wife beater to alcoholic, bar fighter to chain smoker, he was a professional at slow suicide. He ate like a death row inmate on his last meal and took every drug known to man. My dad was like a plane crash survivor everyday --lucky to be alive.

My entire young life revolved the habits he paraded daily. The ones I grew to despise. He had three sisters and seven brothers; all in the grave before him. All of them before the age of fifty. He remained one of three "Bunch's" alive. His brother and me. He was 48-years-old at the time of his stroke. I wasn't even 20.

This isn't a "woe is me" story, it's the opposite. I want everyone to know my motivation, not just my experience. Experience is the reason you should keep listening, motivation is the reason you should keep reading.

When it comes to the life changing habits described in this book, you can rest assured it wasn't just to look cute on the beach. It's not just because I wanted to hit a white ball farther.

Selfishly, I wanted more time with my dad. I never wanted anyone to feel as helpless, selfish, and worthless as I did the day I entered that hospital room. Even if the person in the bed deserved what they were getting or not. And let me get this out right now, my dad deserved it and so do you and so do I if we don't choose to be better.

That's my motivation, the rest is my experience.

Young Me:
If you think I'd trade my broken home childhood for one with more hugs and kisses and less syringes and limes, you'd be wrong.

I can't thank our creator enough for giving me an example of how NOT to be. Exactly how NOT to treat others. Exactly how NOT to love women. Exactly how NOT to eat. I was gifted a front row seat to a really good horror flick. It's called, "How NOT to Live."

"And let me get this out right now, my dad deserved it and so do you and so do I if we don't choose to be better."

No, I wouldn't trade that for the world. Nor should you expect me to. It's you, the reader who I wish to benefit heavily from what superficially appears as misfortune. I believe it's my obligation to pass those blessing on to you.

Since my dad was hardly around, I replaced him with fast food and I got fat. Since my mom had to work around the clock to support her and I, she left me with a TV babysitter and chocolate friends. And I love her dearly for it. She did what she had to, just as my father did. They made me who I am.

I envied the muscular dudes in movies and loved bodybuilding. I wanted to look like a comic book hero not the fat kid from "Goonies." Thankfully, at least by the time I entered high school, I was as obsessive as a toddler with a new toy. With obsession comes one question I can't stop asking and never answer: "Is this the best life has, is this the best way to get what I want?" If you're reading this, I bet you say the same things.

The day I turned 18 I joined a gym. I was completely ignorant, knew fitness would take time and body-sculpting wouldn't happen overnight, but I still thought I could "figure fitness out fast" and achieve Arnold-Abs, Superman-pecs, and a Batman-back before I was 20.

I'm 35-years-old and I do have a chest that enters the room before me, but it's no Superman (he was an alien and steel after all). But the process has taught me novels of information and I'm still learning everyday

I've read everything, tried everything, and pestered everyone bigger and better and older than me. At 19 I started personal training so I could live within the sea of treadmills, mirrors and spandex.

I thought I was the the Sultan of fitness until my dad went all stroke-victim on me. It's not like he was winning beauty pageants or Superbowl's before that, but his fall painted a masterpiece even Michelangelo would've been proud of. I felt like the fog of my youth had burnt off giving way to the afternoon of my future and it wasn't arms the size of cannons or tree trunk legs; it was health. I wanted to live well and I wanted it for my friends.

Enter CrossFit
I found CrossFit eight years ago.

Until that day I felt like a Dolphin in a net. I could see freedom, but I couldn't swim in it.

CrossFit set me free.

CrossFit is functional movement performed at the utmost of intensity in a variety of ways. Meaning, today's workout looks very different from yesterday, boredom is eliminated by variety, and results are guaranteed by effort.

CrossFit was created by Greg Glassman, a well-spoken college dropout that you would love to spend every waking moment with. He's one of those guys that makes you want to sit indian style and listen to stories about doing laundry or driving to the store or saving the world. He's our Coach ... our leader. He's a man a community would fight for. A man haters love to hate.

I had no clue what CrossFit was when I found it, but I loved it like a yelping puppy in a box full of mutts.

"CrossFit was created by Greg Glassman, a well-spoken college dropout that you would love to spend every waking moment with. He's one of those guys that makes you want to sit indian style and listen to stories about doing laundry or driving to the store or saving the world. He's our Coach ... our leader. He's a man a community would fight for. A man haters love to hate."

The Plan
Guidance comes to us supernaturally whether we realize it or not.

This book is an expression of what I've learned at the feet of better men and women than myself. It's about how I formed their genius into my own God given capabilities and manufactured a unique philosophy. So unique, in fact, I think that void of all ego, this book could be one of the most important texts you could ever read.

This book tells of how CrossFit saved a guy like me, and how I know it can do the same for you.

The only thing left now is the start. But before you turn the page give-up on everything you thought was correct. This book is good, but it's not going to change a mind dead set against its teaching. If you've bought it so you can tear it apart then I'll save you the trouble. However, if you're ready for something new, then turn the page without expectation or argument, and watch what happens.

CHAPTER 1

THE RX

If you don't care about the "why," this chapter is for you. You probably skip to the end of movies and Game of Thrones too, don't you?

1. Mark your calendar thirty days from now. Then forty five. The RX is a 30 day program at least. Forty-five days is better. Once you have made it that long ... why stop? This isn't a fad, it's a lifestyle.
2. Take pictures of yourself every Monday. Use good lighting from lots of angles.
3. Take these measurements:
   Waist
   Hips
   Thigh
   Body-fat
   Weight
   Blood Pressure
   Triglyceride
   HDL
   LDL
   Fasting Blood Glucose
   H1ac
   C-reactive protein
   Vitamin D

4. Empty your cupboards and rearrange your house. Little changes don't work, and old scenery reminds us of bad habits. Make sure all the bad food is out of the house and all the bad attitudes are out of your life.
5. Stop eating all grains. Stop all Dairy. Stop all legumes. Stop all alcohol. Stop all fruit. Stop all sugar.
6. Start eating only; Meats, nuts, seeds, veggies, coconut, ghee, and water.
7. Increase your fat intake until you're not hungry after a meal for at least five hours.
8. Start CrossFitting at a CrossFit affiliate at least three times a week. The support system will keep you honest. Diet doesn't work alone, neither does exercise for that matter.
9. Sleep. At least eight hours a night.
10. Avoid almost all carbohydrate. Except those found in nuts and veggies.
11. Journal your results and report back to yourself and your supporters often. Give it some time before remeasuring as slower than anticipated results often derail even the strongest followers. If you have been unhealthy for years, it won't come back in days.
12. Drink water.

Well there is the present without having to put the cookies out and wait for Santa. You can dive in on these imperative twelve steps without ever studying the "why" in the following chapters. However, when the questions come and self doubt meanders in, the answers in those chapters may get your through those tough times.

CHAPTER 2

WHY LISTEN TO ME?

Nobody window shops healthy. Healthy is a purchase we buy at the proportion in which we lose it. Usually, unsuccessfully.

The guy sitting in front of me is fat, he's not the only fat guy that will sit in front of me today. Mark, a cog in the fitness machine, a contract, a tenant to a rent seeking fitness center. He's the hundredth, or thousandth--I can't remember anymore--membership that I've sold.

His robust cheeks are Baptist-preacher red. If he had a beard, and was more jolly, he'd be Santa. Does Santa have high-blood pressure? Hypertensive is what the smart people call it ... simple folks like me call it motivation.

"So you're saying if I sign this, you're going to help me get in shape?," Mark asked.

Before we go on, did you see the episode of The Simpsons where Homer gained nearly 100 lb. so he could go on disability? Well, add 50 lb.

Mark's divorced, has kids and makes a lot of jokes about himself and politics, a lot of big folks do. He's also a newly diagnosed diabetic. A doctor ordered fitness rookie. The only difference between this guy and every other fat guy I thought I could save with a monthly gym payment was his next question.

"If this place is going to help me, why hasn't it helped you?," he asked.

The small office we were in had a big mirror on the wall. It gives the room an illusion of bigness. Without saying a word I looked. My reflection was no illusion. Who was selling who the membership now?

"Healthy is a purchase we buy at the proportion in which we lose it. Usually, unsuccessfully."

At the time I was trying to be a competitive bodybuilder. Some competitive bodybuilders stay in shape all year long, but the majority have an offseason. To most competitive bodybuilders offseason means they workout all the time and eat whatever they want; chicken, vegetables, coconut, ... ice cream, pizza, Reese's.

"I'm in the offseason," I said with a poker face. Back then he was a sell, and a sell is a sell. ABC, right? I imagined myself snatching him out of that chair and twisting him up like an MMA fighter.

"Oh, does that mean I get an offseason from being healthy too?," he asked.

My stomach played tug-o-war and I paused like I was praying. Like never before, I questioned myself.

Mark was the most honest man I'd ever met. He was my inciting incident and that's what I want this book to be for you.

An inciting incident is that thing in movies that makes the main character "DO." Maybe they decide to finally go to college or buy an engagement ring.

Maybe they finally call their long lost father. The double "I" is beyond scene one and it's the reason we keep watching the movie.

Are you happy with your story?

Mark wasn't and I wasn't either. Inciting incidents happen everyday, we just ignore most of them.

"My goal isn't health today, maybe later," I said. "My today goal is to get as big as possible, so that when it's time to cut down and compete on stage I'm as muscular as possible."

That was the first time I had ever said that out loud. I hated the way it sounded. Still do.

Without health, everything else is just luck.

"I see," he said.

Please, don't ask, I repeated in my head.

"How many times have you competed?," he asked.

It's not everyday that you're confronted with the lies you tell yourself. It's like another author reading your book and tearing it apart right before your eyes. Here I was, fat, being torn apart by a fatter man I was selling health to.

Health can't be sold. Health can't be bought.

"I haven't completed yet, I'm not big enough," I said.

Bruised, I managed to change the subject back to Mark, his divorce and those kids he was surely about to leave Fatherless.

"Where do I sign?," Mark finally asked.

Despite my hypocritical rhetoric, he took a chance. I didn't sell him anything other that a double standard and we both knew that.

"Without health, everything else is just luck."

Bodybuilding, Drugs, Food, Addiction:
I've lived in a gym since I was 16-years-old. I'm 35.

I love the way superheroes and Schwarzenegger's look. They remind me of moral codes and a right way to do everyday activities. I began working out because I wanted to be like them ... I still do.

The first fitness membership I purchased was in Maryville, Tennessee. The guy who gave me a tour looked like a baseball player not the bodybuilder I wanted to be. He showed me the pretty machines upstairs and explained the saunas and showers on the second level (and is it just me or do old people get way too comfortable with being naked?).

After that we hit the racquetball courts and aerobics room. *Cute.*

We finally hit a green metal door. The corners were rusted and it didn't close all the way. The light creeping through was different too, a country road on a fall morning

"Here's the basement," my tour guide said.

As soon as he opened it I thought I was back in junior high on the rubber mat wrestling, getting pinned by the guy who sweats really bad and is as slippery as a non-stick pan. There must be a pool that he hasn't showed me yet either because right now my eyes are burning from the chlorine; everything reminds me of week old socks and burnt tires.

He walks past mounds of iron and rusted dumbbells, strew about like casualties because they're too big for racks. I can hear metal clanging as rhythmically as a heartbeat. The elevator music that was background noise everywhere else has been exchanged for Judas Priest.

He stops before we round the last corner. "Let me show you the pool," he says turning around. "I don't swim," I said and kept on moving forward.

The rubber floor ended, I was walking on dirt staring at a group of very big men lifting things I'd dreamed of, looking like the hero's I wanted to be. "I'm cool right here man, thanks," I said ending the tour.

For the next month or so, they ignored me except for the occasional "humph," meaning move or be moved. Since the only guys who trained in the basement were black, I almost asked if they wanted me to leave because I was white. But more than anything I wanted to join their group like I wanted to touch boobs. They wanted to train.

I set-up stations within ear-shot. Whatever they did worked and I figured, since they weren't talking to me, I could at least eavesdrop. After they left I repeated what they'd done. Back then my total gym time was no less than three hours everyday - spying, and training.

Eight weeks after I began, while I was making dumbbell flys look like seizures, Doc eclipsed the light above me. "Let me show you something," he said.

Doc was the biggest black man in a room full of black men and I was the smallest, and whitest, child in a room full of heroes.

My hands began to sweat and I remembered someone tying a really tight tie around my neck. A comic book superhero was standing over me offering advice. I probably looked like Ralphie on the Christmas Story when his dad said he still had one present left. It was 30-seconds at best and it meant the world to me. It still does.

Doc wore glasses and carried himself like men do. I thought back to the teachers I had respected most while I was in high school, how they managed to show confidence when they taught people things. Younger people. They seemed to lose that confidence anytime they were taken out of that environment. Doc was someone who commanded respect no matter where he was or who he talked to. He walked like he was made of steel with a chest that entered the room a full second before the rest of him.

I never thought it was my place to initiate the conversation with my betters so I let him do all the work. Over the weeks he showed me more and I managed to say thanks and ask a question or two. His crew kinda side eyed his actions every time we talked, but they would never dare challenge Doc. He was their leader. He was the most commanding even though he talked the least.

Doc was the biggest black man in a room full of black men and I was the smallest, and whitest, child in a room full of heroes.

The day I finally benched with Doc and his crew ranks right up there with graduating high school. It was like one life ending so a better one can begin. I remember him leading me into four men that would block out the sun if we were outside. Here I was, 5' 8", 150 lb. Their shortest crew member was over six-foot, their lightest over 230 lb. I thought they would hate and laugh at me.

I reached ... it was like holding a slab of meat to wild dogs ... I thought a nub would come back.

Huge tooth filled grins, the ones where you see the teeth in the back, shined. They all shook my hand and patted me on the back. I don't remember what I benched, I don't remember much of anything except this: I felt like I belonged, and that felt better than anything had before.

After we finished, Doc took me out to his car.

"What are you taking," he asked.

"Taking?," I repeated. "Yeah, supplements ya know, taking," he said. "Ohhhh, well," I procrastinated.

"Here, let me show you," Doc said.

His trunk looked like GNC. He pulled out a big jug, a medium jug, and a little jug. He gave me directions on how to take them. I never looked at the labels and took every last drop of the parking lot supplements I got from the trunk of a man named Doc. A friend I will never forget.

⋏

When we're young and sometimes when we're not, vanity is our motivation for everything.

That changes the day disaster strikes and we discover our own mortality. Health, then, becomes more important than looks. Fortunately, pleasing aesthetics is a side effect of great health.

Still, I spent a long time working out for the mirror, much of which made me healthier, and I learned a few tricks that can't be forgotten, some not worth the time, and others so dangerous I should whoop my own ass for even trying them

Here's a taste:

- Carbs don't give you energy. At least not the energy you want.
- Fat does not make you fat. At least, not how "they" say it does.

- Food is an addiction and a necessity.
- Addiction can be overcome.
- Exercise should be brief.
- Carbs are population control.
- Many people already know all of the above.
- Many people who know don't care.
- Facts and examples cannot overcome an emotional and irrational mind.
- The body's defense system is the mind.
- The mind is the source for success.
- The mind is the source for failure.
- Carbs are voluntary servitude through food.
- The food pyramid was purchased, not created. He who had the most dollars, not he who had the right answer.
- Supplements are a business, not a solution.
- Fish oil works, so does Vitamin D.
- Doctors lie because we want them to.
- Most of us can't handle honesty.
- Your friends can be your greatest enemies; family your greatest obstacle.
- The relationships you create and nurture either destroy you, or propel you.
- Community is the best health you can dream of.
- Men and Women will die for points.
- Women are stronger than men.
- Change is pain. Pain scars. Life sucks without scars.
- Without breaking yourself there's no chance to rebuild better than before.
- Successful workouts are social.
- Suffering is life and your ability to grow from it is exactly related to life's achievements.
- Your ability to be comfortable when being made uncomfortable is worth its weight in gold.
- Kids smell hypocrisy, adults wear it like cologne.

- Jealousy prevents victory more than any other emotion.
- Forgiveness is the road to salvation.

Bodybuilding is a gateway drug:
The life of a competitive bodybuilder is selfish, ruled by the clock, food and iron. No other sport requires adherence in quite so many domains. It's about water, drugs, food, training, sleep and more. It's about the edge; that special thing that works especially well for you.

I worked a long time to find the edge and here's some of what I learned:

- Eating six to eight meals per day is totally unnecessary. Supplement manufactures and fast restaurant dining came up with this so we would consume the 4000+ calories created per human per day.
- You CAN eat too much protein, but it won't kill you or wreck your kidney's, you just get fat.
- Work the entire body as often as possible. Bodybuilders injure easily because they train body parts independently.
- Workouts are sprints, not marathons.
- Cardio just burns Calories; most of us want to burn fat.
- Off seasons are for quitters. There is never a season where I want to be less healthy.

For years I ate every two or three hours and took fancy oils, shakes and powders. I read magazines, physician's desk references, and updated pharmacy manuals. I even hired multiple trainers and browsed the internet for anything that could make me gain one more ounce of awesome.

I learned a lot ... the hard way.

In a few short years I rose naturally from 155 lb. to just over 200 lb. All with shakes, chicken and whatever else that was loaded with Calories to make me look like my heroes. But that wasn't enough.

Juice:

I knew I would become a human pin cushion the day I picked up my first barbell. Steroids and the propaganda that surrounded them didn't scare me, in fact it made me want them more. Still, if there's such a thing, I wanted to do drugs the right way.

I studied for two years before I jammed my first needle in my right butt cheek. By the time I finally thought I knew all there was to know, I could have taught a college course on testosterone.

The icy touch of hypothermia is all I remember. I was standing, pants half pulled down, mooning no-one in particular for two hours. I held that first needled a centimeter from my skin and just stared at it, gripping the dresser with my free hand. Sweat puddled the ground, my tough guy exterior melted into the carpet. I asked God to let me be big … big and alive.

I wasn't scared of the pain, I was scared of the consequences. Did my muscle bound pharmacist sell me motor oil? What if I hit an artery? What if I passed out and my roommate came home and found me with a shelf full of Class Three Controlled Substances - my roommate the Christian?

In the end the want for more muscle overcame intelligence and I plunged 1 cc of oil in it my rear.

I didn't die. And, it worked.

Over the years I progressed from "regular" drugs purchased at strip clubs and gyms to homemade brews from cow pellets. I even tried a version of rat poison that can cook organs from the inside out - twice.

All for vanity.

I gained muscle, of course, but also fat and water. My weight soared from just over two-bills to nearly 260 lb. at my most imposing.

At 5' 8" 260 lb., breathing is exhausting, stairs are terrifying and tying your shoes is a dream. But I was big and strong and nothing else mattered.

"I knew I would become a human pin cushion the day I picked up my first barbell."

By the time I started my fifth cycle I was addicted. It wasn't a high or low I was after, steroids don't work that way, it was the results.

Steroids are the reward man gives himself, I argued for years. They don't make training or eating well any less necessary, they reward you that much more for putting in the work. And since I loved the work, I became addicted to the extra reward.

With drugs came the courage to compete and the roller coaster of offseason and game time. On stage I was 180 lb. and 5-percent body fat. The day after that I was 20-pounds heavier.

And so it went, drugs, big, drugs, small, drugs, big, drugs, insane. The amounts I took weren't so much damaging to the body as they were to my self-esteem. Imagine every girl on the planet drooling over you one day, ignoring you the next.

Steroids were never the problem, the extremist behavior they brought out in me were. That's what steroids do; they make you more of who you already are, and for a guy like me, that's scary as hell.

That's the real reason you shouldn't take steroids. Not some bullshit public service announcement, but cold hard truth from a guy that lived it for years. Not because some dumbass doctor with diabetes and a potbelly says they're unhealthy, but because you start loving the version of you on them, and hating the version of you off them.

Am I sorry I took them? No. I know more about them than just about everyone. And that knowledge will save people from making the same mistakes

I made. People that may have otherwise been unable to cope with the depression of withdrawal, the loss of muscle, of confidence.

Today, if any young athletes asks me if they should take steroids, I can honest say HELL NO!

Not because your liver will fail, your heart will explode or your kidneys will pop, but because you'll fall in love with whoever you are while you take them, and when it comes time to stop, you might not be able to let go.

"That's what steroids do; they make you more of who you already are, and for a guy like me, that's scary as hell."

Thankfully, when I needed saving the most, CrossFit was there for me. Without it I'm not sure I'd be here today. CrossFit saved me. CrossFit saves everyone. From the day I discovered CrossFit, the hardest drug I've done is caffeine.

Thanks Coach.

Enter CrossFit:
"Josh, you gotta see this!"

Wipers, the clip read. The athlete, while hanging from a pull-up bar, body parallel to the ground, moved his legs from side to side--like a windshield wiper. The clip was gritty with offensive music. I loved it.

"I can do that," I said sprinting to the bar. My half-assed attempt left my ego damaged and my soul craving more.

It was 2007 and I spent the night diving into CrossFit.

The next day I tried "Fran". A hallmark CrossFit workout that mixed Gymnastics and weightlifting, consisting of 21-15-9 reps or 95 lb. thrusters and pull-ups.

Before I began, surrounded by a sea of machines in the fitness center I worked at for years, I thought of how cool it will be to crush this 90 rep romp called a workout. After all, 95 lb. and pull-ups are easy ...right?

That's where things kind get hazy, I remember looking at the ceiling 12-minutes later. My forearms felt "odd" (by odd I mean they felt like watermelons were growing within them). My skin was so tight over I thought they would burst and I felt something in my lungs I had never felt, I think it's called acid and it burns.

After that I could have argued a million reasons why CrossFit wouldn't work. All lies to cover up insecurity. CrossFit crushed me and I loved it for that and always have. A little crushing is exactly what we need more of.

"Fran" showed me how sick I really was. Right then I chose CrossFit.

The day after my first CrossFit workout, I decided to open an affiliate.

I didn't bandwagon CrossFit because of money. It certainly wasn't because it was easy or bright and shiny like some turnkey franchise. It was because everything Coach said was true. It was because everything coach said I'd said before. It was simple, meaningful, and most of all, it meant I wasn't crazy. I love that man for who he is, everything he's given, everything he's taught me.

The next day I met my employer of seven years, the guy who owned the gym I trained at. I was the dashing young graduate with future in his eyes. He was the wise mentor who will clearly see the opportunity in what I am about to present.

It reminds me of the first Mother's Day present I bought with my own money; a candle--vanilla I think. I was so proud when I gave it to her that I could hardly let her unwrap it.

"A little crushing is exactly what we need more of."

This man wasn't just a boss, he was a friend. We spent Christmas together, birthdays, regular days. Surely he would be supportive, especially since CrossFit is like apples are to oranges when it comes regular gyms and CrossFit boxes. They both have weights and people, but that's about all they share.

"I'm opening a CrossFit," I said to my boss. At the time, I had no startup money or location, or anything really. "What's CrossFit?," he asked.

About four minutes later, after a silly explanation because I really didn't know either, he just kinda said "OK".

And I didn't just tell him, I asked him to be my partner.

He fired me the the next day.

Looking back, I couldn't be more thankful. He was that voice of can't I had to overcome. He became my 9th grade Spanish teacher who said I would never amount to anything. To prove her wrong, I mastered another language and brought an "F" to the highest "A" out of spite. Now, if I failed, I would have to ask for my job back. I would have to ask a friend, who really wasn't a friend, if I could work for him again. I wasn't going to let that happen.

I wrote a double-spaced thirty-three page business plan that night. It took me less than three hours. After that my brother and I, who was also my business partner, started asking for money.

Have you ever felt like God had a plan for you but everyone else was against you? That's how I felt after the 6th bank turned us down.

At the 7th bank my brother and I prayed. We had prayed before, but this one was different. It seemed more real, like we were really speaking to a third party who wanted us to keep going.

My brother is a Doctor of Pharmacy. He's two years younger than me and well liked at parties. He's one of those quippy one-liner guys who makes people smile and feel comfortable. If he was in a horror movie he'd be the guy next to the main character you would hope lives through the entire flick.

He's the kind of man who sticks up for the little guy. My younger brother, a man I admire more than he knows. A man that after graduating college at ONU (Ohio Northern University) had faith enough to put his credit on the line for a business neither of us knew anything about. My brother never loses faith in me.

As I presented my case to the seventh banker I noticed how clean his desk was. How see-thru the window was behind him, the one that lead to a cornfield.

The bank was a "farming" bank. Our last chance. I couldn't focus on the guy sitting across from me. I felt like I had a fever. Looking back, I think it's because I was trying to be someone I wasn't. I was trying to present a business when I hate business more than anything.

I got up and took of my suit jacket. It didn't fit anyway, they never do when you don't have a tailor and you workout a lot.

"I wrote that plan in three hours," I said. The banker was kinda shocked. "I have no real experience to speak of, but I think we can help people, and at the very least I think we will help enough people to get you your money back with interest. Isn't that what you want to hear?" I asked.

"You don't own a home, and have virtually no collateral," he said.

"Yup, and my brother's school loans are over $200,000, and we're crazy for even asking. Oh, and we're in our mid-twenties. We're a huge risk. But it will work."

"You need to come in and sign some papers to start an account with us, then we can deposit your money," my voicemail said two days later. I felt like it was the first time I had taken a breath in a month, the end of the roller coaster feeling when you realize you made it. We all made it.

My brother didn't answer his phone when I called to deliver the news. I waited until he got home and told him since we lived together anyway. He was happy for me. He called it hustling. "I have been educated, and I follow the rules, and for that I will be rewarded in a certain way," he said. "But you, you're a hustler and you will be rewarded because you don't stop"

Two days after "Mr. Banker" for the 7th time, we had $40k burning a hole in a brand new bank account.

Today:
Today, Practice CrossFit, the CrossFit affiliate we began eight years ago, lives in it's third home. Just under 10,000 square-feet of awesomeness. We have seen thousands of pounds lost, and thousands of pull-ups gained. We train CrossFit Games athletes, National Level Weightlifters, Powerlifters, Physique Competitors and more. More than anything, we train people who just want to feel better. And for that, I'm most proud

I've made a lot of mistakes along the way, spent more money than I have, stayed up late worrying about friends, pushed when I should've hugged; It's a life I wouldn't trade for anything, a life i'm proud to live.

If CrossFit saved me--a fat, delusion, addicted, hypocrite--then it will save you.

CHAPTER 3

THE APPROACH

Have you ever noticed how heavy a door feels when you know you're not going to like what's behind it?

The door leading to my apartment sometime ago was one of the heaviest doors I had ever opened. My girlfriend of three years had walked out and that door led straight to lonely.

"God, what am I doing wrong", I shouted. "You're too loud asshole," God said. Bang-Bang-Bang … wait God doesn't punch walls, neighbors do when wall ar as thin as orange peels.

I had become a personal trainer free from all side incomes. I had yet to open a CrossFit, or even hear of it, but I was training a decent number of people that increased everyday. "Why isn't this working….it has to," I repeated to no one.

Back then my best and worst quality was absorbing the failure of others and making it my own. I would beat myself up when my clients failed to meet their goals regardless of their actions. I would hold myself more accountable as opposed to them. I would look for another supplement, exercise, tool, pill.

I couldn't bare that 50-percent of my clients saw incredible results, while the other half left dissatisfied.

I blamed myself.

Finally, after much soul searching, it hit me. Food doesn't keep us down, our minds do.

I realized that the half getting results were mentally ready to change and the other half simply wasn't there yet. The next question became; how do we get ready for change?

Upstairs

I read my athletes everyday. From there I can guide and adjust them based off real world data, not numbers in a book.

On paper the race may look the same to everyone. But once you're running things change. A hill to some is a mountain to others. A warm-up for you is a marathon to me. Realizing this is the first step in an endless race. It means we don't all get there the at the same time, and that's cool.

The chapters to come may appear somewhat random. They are a tapestry woven together over time, not a linear thought.

I believe, and hopefully the book will prove, that for every physical change we experience, there must be a mental adjustment to accompany. Without the mind on board the body will simply never set sail.

The Plan

I've learned a great deal from watching others and I aim to to tell their stories the best I can. I think that's how we learn; by reading about others who are just like us, who have done what we want to do.

I don't claim to have all the answers but I have tried a lot of experiments. I don't presume to know it all, and I'm sure the second edition of this book will argue points in the first. Thats good, thats progress.

If you feel like it's been a long time since you have made any progress, or the path is so foreign you faintly remember it, I invite you to open your mind and dive right in.

CHAPTER 4

CHOOSE BETTER

W hen you boil it down, life is two options:

Choose to be better, or choose to be the same. There is no greater shame than waking up tomorrow the same way you woke up today.

This book is intended to place you as close as possible to the promise land by truth, motivation, cute analogies, real life testimonials and tested triumphs. However, as good as I think this book is, and as meaningful as it can be, it can't open that door for you. Only you can make the choice.

Temptation fills us to be less than we are capable of. To choose to set the bar down, to drop the ball, to wait for the clock instead of work for the clock. Temptation is a gift. Temptation gives us resistance, and resistance makes us stronger.

We were born for better if we choose it.

When we resist being like everyone else, when our choice becomes leaving the old skin behind and adopting the exterior armor of a warrior, we can truly become better today than we were yesterday. Life is really just that simple. Life is just making today better than any day that has come before it.

The ability to recognize the times when these tests, these opportunities, these choices arise has been forever blessed within us. We can comfortably keep our mouth shut fearing the response of speaking the truth. We can remain seated when we know life is begging us to stand and fight. We can pull our chin over that bar for the last time of the day because we know how sweet tomorrow's sunrise will be if we do, and how bitter it will taste if we don't.

No diet in the world will help you during these times. There isn't a supplement for integrity. There isn't a trainer for enlightenment. There is only you and your choice to be better today than yesterday.

CHAPTER 5

WHOLE GRAINS, WHOLE MILK, OH MY

The great frontier I called it. Except there was nothing particularly great about it and it was about as frontierish as any suburban neighborhood with one too many cul-de-sacs and roundabouts.

It's where I grew up, the first real home my mom could afford in a neighborhood where locked doors were a choice, not a must. There was three bedrooms, a big bay window where our Calico lived, and a yard that connected me to others kids in the area.

I remember the three pretty blonds who lived just over the metal fence. I remember Christmas Day target practice with my dad and new bow and arrow. I remember my mom's stomach hurting every other day.

By the time I was 18-years-old and dying to be on my own, I'd forgotten that she spent so many of her days in pain. The selfish and stupid kid that I was just thought it was her lot in life, intestines that hated her. I out and forget.

More than 10 passed. My brother became a doctor and I opened a CrossFit. If my parents didn't like him better already, they sure did after that. Who wants to claim a tatted up son who works out for a living when you have a doctor in the family?

One Christmas, Justin and I drove to visit our parents in Tennessee. We listened to sad songs, remembered the girls we'd lost and talked about the girls we wanted. We made it home by midnight.

The next morning I ransacked the house looking for coffee. What normal human goes a day--an hour--without coffee? My mom, that's who. Apparently I picked up a thing or two while I was away, coffee being one of my better habits.

Her cupboards were full glasses with apples, towels with apples and plates with apples; she likes apples. One shelf, however, wasn't full of apple marked paraphernalia, but pill bottles. More bill bottles than a GNC. Papaya, Ginger, Spirulina; she had everything.

I know my stuff and I know what all of it was for--digestion. I needed coffee.

"What's with all the pills?," I asked that night at dinner.

"There for your stomach," she said. "Remember, mom's stomach hurts a lot."

And now you know my mom. She still talks about herself in third person, talks in a northern accent even though she's lived in the South most her life, tans easily, has fine as cotton hair and lives with the same pain her entire life. Pain I forgot about a long time ago.

Her constant battle came rushing back, and in fact, so did mine. When I was young my stomach was sensitive. Not as bad as mom--I wasn't bedridden three or more days a week--but I was out for the count multiple times a month. For some reason, it just stopped.

Mom's didn't.

"I didn't remember until just now," I said. "It's been like that all this time?"

"It's a little better with the supplements," she said.

After that, she passed the garlic bread. Ironic?

"Mom, remember that Paleo diet I've told you about?," ...

For years I'd explained Paleo to my mom and for years she paid me as much attention as a housewife watching her kid do another cannonball at the public pool. But this time was different. This time my brother, the doctor, was sitting right beside me.

"It's what I do," my brother chimed in after I was done explaining.

"You do!"

It was the best Christmas present ever. Proof that even your own mother could care less about your experience, unless it's doctor approved.

Three weeks after Christmas, I called to check in.

"I'm down 22 lb.," she said. I was just calling to check in. The day after Christmas she began Paleo and didn't stop.

"And my stomach hasn't hurt since."

My mom never goes to the doctor. She's never had her stomach officially diagnosed with anything. Officially, I can't place blame, but unofficially, I have my suspicions ...

Celiac Sucks:
Celiac Syndrome or Celiac Sprue is the name given when certain side effects are demonstrated after consuming Gluten. CS damages the gut lining or villa

preventing nutrients from being absorbed, therefore offering a host of other problems.

Gluten Primer

Gluten is a protein found in wheat, most cereal grains, pastas, desserts and just about everything at the bottom of the food pyramid. We all have an aversion of some sort to it. Some of us just demonstrate our sensitivity differently.

Gluten containing foods:

Barley, including barley malt
Bran
Bulgur
Couscous
Farina
Kamut
Orzo
Semolina
Spelt
Tabbouli
Wheat
Semolina
Farina
Cake
Bread
Cupcakes
Tortillas
Bagels
Sandwich buns
Hotdog buns
Pizza crust

Some of these are redundant but I wanted those who are truly unaware the gravity at which we make gluten a staple in the average human's diet.

The most heinous of offenders are mentioned above. A quick google search is much better at telling you exactly what out right contains Gluten or what may have similar effects for one reason or another.

In short, Gluten is the stuff that makes breads absorb water giving it a more palatable texture. Without it, bread would be putty. Gluten also absorbs gases to help breads rise and it's the reason pastry's and such go stale.

When Celiacs Sufferers Eat Gluten:
While a gluten allergy may send someone into anaphylactic shock and kill them like right now, gluten intolerance doesn't. At least not immediate death, but death is death no matter how you cut it.

When someone with CS eats a burger - bun and all - they tear at the lining of their stomach. This of course could cause erratic digestion issue like gas, diarrhea, or constipation. But lets say it doesn't. Let's say it does something we may not attribute to food in the least.

"And my stomach hasn't hurt since."

What if that bad food shows up as a reddish face, fatigue, decreased appetite, weight gain or joint pain. Does this sound like you after eating your favorite plate of pasta or morning bowl of cereal? Doesn't that sound like just about everyone after they eat gluten containing grains long enough?

As it stands, one-percent of Americans are diagnosed Celiac sufferers. It's estimated that 66-percent are just undiagnosed. People like my mom.

Autoimmune is suicide not disease
Celiacs is autoimmune. Autoimmune disorders are malfunctions within us that make "normal" or "domestic" parts of us look "abnormal" or "foreign". And if you haven't noticed it yet, your body is prejudice. If anything looks

like a Muslim flying a hijacked 747, it's attacked without restraint. This in-air protection is a valuable evolution.

Autoimmune disorders are too vast to be covered, too common to be ignored, and easily avoided. We may very well have a genetic predisposition to Celiacs, but as discussed before, the children of alcoholics are predisposed to be drunks, but they still gotta drink. Celiacs suffers still gotta eat gluten to get sick.

Unfortunately, autoimmune disorders are never outgrown like allergies, hence why celiacs is a forever kinda cold, not a gazuntite. But while we can't cure this autoimmune reaction, we can control our drugs (food).

Crohn's Disease, and Ulcerative Colitis:

CD, and UC are not to be forgotten, and I'm sure if you have been diagnosed with either you never will. While celiacs has its offender - Gluten, CD and UC, on the surface appear less simple.

While it may be true, various sufferers have afflictions resulting from a smorgasbord of foods, it's not hard to leap headfirst into each diet and find a few huge consistent needles in the haystack.

CD, and UC are autoimmune also. Sufferers have chronic inflammation of the gastrointestinal tract caused by any number of offending foods.

For an autoimmune disease to kick in we have to be born with it, then we have to trigger it by eating certain foods that will probably always hurt us.

The Paleo diet is not only void of all irritants and allergens; grains, legumes, dairy, soy, nightshades, and more, but it provides ample nutrients and a prime gastrointestinal playground for those nutrients to be absorbed, not depleted or attacked.

I'm cool, I have a cast-iron stomach

If I could bewitch the planet into following Paleo like a religion I would. If I could mesmerize the world into giving up grains, dairy, legumes, while eating only meats, nuts, seeds, veggies and coconuts, without even knowing why...I would. However, since I'm rather poor at black magic, I'll just keep giving you the facts.

Even if you're a card carrying, hot wing eating, beer drinking dairy farmer without a stomach ache on record, I guarantee you are still crippled by allergens and toxins found in modern day foods. And I'm not referring to the obvious like sugar and tequila. I'm talking the food pyramid's whole grains, dairy, legumes, even eggs.

It is imperative you leave out the suicidal food for the entire 30 day life changing challenge we'll describe later. The simple difference in how you will feel is more of a sales-pitch than I could ever give you, and realistically, I don't make anything for you avoiding things like grains, and dairy. You already bought my book. What I tell you comes from the heart of someone helping, and the mind of someone who has tried it, and every other way imaginable.

Grains if you don't have CS, IBS, UC, or the like

Grains grown all over the planet sustain life at a fraction of the cost of cattle. That alone should make you question whether they're at the bottom of the food pyramid for health or profit.

Grains like oats, wheat, barley, buckwheat, quinoa, rye and more have been around for a paltry thousands years compared to a humans rather long stint on this little berg we all enjoy so much. And there lies the first problem. We are not used to them yet.

The grain grass or seed contains layers. Germ, bran, endosperm. This is great for the grain, but not so much for anything consuming it. These layers serve as defense systems to animals consuming an otherwise nutritious food source.

Lectins

A lectin is a glycoprotein contained in grains, dairy and legumes. A Lectin protein does not break down like other proteins into simple aminos. Lectins hideout attached to your gut wall until they decide to punch their way through entering your circulatory system, whole, undigested, intact.

After Lectins have entered circulation your "body-guard" - the immune system - tries to heal your gut lining. Second, the immune system signals an alert to the defense set up "Kill the lectin"...but what the troops here is, "kill the traitor". Remember Lectin isn't the odd man out, he looks like everybody else, and when you can't find "the bad muslim" you hunt "all muslims"

Eventually your immune system bodyguard finds the lectin demon looking like all its friend. Without discrimination your body guard kills them all, and when you immune system attacks its healthy self, you're officially autoimmune.

Phytates

If the Lectin story wasn't enough to keep even us supposed healthy folks away from grains and the like forever, maybe anti-nutrients will be the kicker.

Phytates are anti-nutrients. Nutrients are good. Anti good means bad... simple.

Particularly, phytates are anti-minerals. When we consume phytates within grains the phytates remain active and bind to other nutrients entering the system. Once phytates bind with a nutrient it can't be absorbed. Not only does it go undigested, but now, after the lectin explosion, and gut deterioration, we have nutrient deficiency to worry about.

This is exactly how things like Vitamin D deficiencies arise. This is how otherwise unheard of diseases twenty five years ago are prevalent today. This is why we take a calcium supplement for an osteo-whatever, that makes everything worse, when we should be absorbing that calcium better by not eating phytates that make it impossible.

But what about fermenting:
An old standard of grain alcohol and bean and vegetable production is "soaking," or "fermenting." Things like wine and kimchi rot and taste better. However, sprouts, oats and just about all seed like grains can be soaked and supposedly improved.

Soaking can lessen the effect of the protease inhibitors and even reduce phytic acid....a little. While more is better in terms of soaking and fermenting. And yes fermenting may enhance good gut bacteria, it still does not eliminate the offending agents, it just makes them more misdemeanor than felony.

I would leave fermenting and soaking to the tree huggers, and just avoid the toxic food hornets nest all together. While a 36-hour soak, or prolonged fermentation may reduce some of the negative, it doesn't automatically lead to a positive.

A dairy disaster, bean blasphemy, and naughty nightshades:
I fought for all these facts to be untrue, just as you may be doing right now. But I experimented on myself and others and the results were undeniable.

I didn't want to believe I was lied to and taken advantage of. I didn't want to believe my favorite foods were really just that bad. That consuming one piece of bread could hurt me for over two weeks.

But fat, acne, hair loss, weak bones, under-active thyroids, cancers, irritable bowels are enough motivation to try anything once. We simply deserve better.

I can't count the number of times I've heard, "I feel all congested after I drink milk, but I love it". I used to say it too, but if you read that again it's like saying "the bullet hurts, but I like the big bang". It's an early warning system. It's the tornado alarm before the funnel, the lighthouse before the rocks. Yet because it's acceptable, because its tradition we forge ahead ignoring the warning until we run ashore and blow out our hull.

As described above legumes, nightshades and dairy contain lectins and many of the same offenders as grains. But even if that wasn't the case, it wouldn't ever make sense to drink calories ... unless your goal is biggest human on the block Ignored calories in beverages accounts for much of the weight gain in America today. That 500 calorie big gulp with that 1000 calorie whopper makes for an odd formation. Try to eat 1500 calories from just nuts...you can't.

Furthermore, dairy is one of the most insulinogenic substances known to man. It's not about an immediate spike of insulin with milk, it's about a prolonged elevated experience we do not recover well from.

Where can I go from here, what can I eat from breakfast, why are you doing this to me?
First give this thirty days and you will be thankful beyond measure. But to get you started try these five "today steps"

1. Begin a journal with your day one pictures. Log how you feel and when. This will be very important as you will see the valley you go to and feel the peak you come out on.
2. Convert your friends. If you try radical behavior alone you need to be radically strong. If you're not the a loner able to discipline yourself, you need friends. I did.
3. Never become hungry. By far and away it is better to overeat quality recommended foods, than to under eat toxic food.
4. Read the don't eat breakfast chapter, then don't eat breakfast.
5. Get your blood-work. The biomarkers in this book are your new bathroom scales

Twelve Step, and eye openers.

For years I taught that diet maintenance included a "variety day". A once a week 24-hour period where all bets were off, and we ate whatever we wanted. But I felt guilty prescribing it, and I felt guilty doing it. I threw away cheat days once and for all years ago, after some friends and I shared a weekend together, friends that listened to me preach about diet.

The game was over and we relaxed, a group of thirteen competitors and me entered our tour bus ready for the 14-hour trip home. We could recover and laugh together ... we could eat.

While sitting on the bus I remembered my alcoholic father. I thought back to the days when he used to rush home from work excited to see the bottle he cared for so much.

"Hi, son," he'd say on his way to the cupboards above the refrigerator.

He would drink until he would run out then go buy more. If we were lucky he would pass out, if we weren't, he'd kill a bottle of Ny-quil three-seconds after a bottle of Southern Comfort. I know addiction.

For several weeks my fellow competitors had been diet diligent. Mostly weighing and measuring, packing their food remaining on the Paleo reservation. They plotted their course, a goal with an end in mind. Now that the goal was reached they seemed to think the journey was over.

I watched as a previously dedicated hoard of athletes told tales of what they wanted to eat. What was most important to their world. I watched, silent, condemning myself for creating such addiction. For suppressing an urge instead of curing it.

The only stop we made was a Flying-J's. It's like a bar with fuel and showers. I used the restroom and returned to the RV and ate my turkey and nuts like it was every other day. My friends didn't.

When they climbed the four stairs into our tight quarters, they had gas station pizza, candy bars, hot wings and everything else they had been denied. Some athletes entered with things they had not consumed in years simply because they could ... just because the door was open.

Smiles dawned their faces like children at Christmas. Like a human watching a train wreck that I created, I couldn't take my eyes off. I was crushed, silent, realizing I had cured nothing with my prescription of weekly variety days. I achieved little more than the suppression of addiction. And addiction suppression is not freedom.

When alcoholics enter the 12-step they're not given a "free" day where they can binge drink. They must stay committed. They are there, after all, to cure addiction, not suppress it. Those serious about cure, about health and change follow the rules. They eliminate the very thing that held them so tight. They solve the problem.

Eventually my fellow competitors passed out and left me to my thoughts. Had I really been so wrong? Was I doing harm?

I'm grateful for that day. I learned that for most of us incorporating a variety day are fighting a battle we'll lose, it's just a matter of time.

The hard sell
I believe we are all searching for a way to eliminate one, if not all of our many vices. I believe the day I stumbled upon the Paleo diet I was well on

my way to curing many of mine. Most of which are not even directly related with food.

It would be great to tell you that you can freely live Paleo 80-percent of the time like many other books will promote, but I can't. It's like giving a child a cigarette to play with instead of a gun.

I'm sure some of us could get away with a glorious life filled with "mostly paleo", and if that is to be your lot then experiment away accepting only some of the curative properties the Paleo diet provides.

Thirty days is long enough to experience many of the goods things Paleo has to offer, but it's not long enough to be cured of the desire or the addiction to food. I recommend pursuing a blameless paleo existence until you have absolutely no desire for sweets, pastas breads or the like. Until you no longer crave that one day of debauchery. Until you could take it or leave it, because it really doesn't matter.

Then and only then can you experience freedom. Maybe you're at a wedding and you enjoy some champagne. Maybe it's thanksgiving and you want to spend time with family. If you're cured you can do this, if you're addicted it's a matter of time before suppression becomes full blown expression.

Freedom from addiction means you don't have to worry about repeating old habits or past mistakes. If we're always looking to that free day for fun, we're not free, we're preparing for a fall.

CHAPTER 6

BUDDHISTS ARE THE BOMB

"And so there is no reason for you to think that any man has lived long because he has grey hairs or wrinkles; he has not lived long—he has existed long."

- Seneca

"So what did you read since our last meeting?," he asked.

This was the we started every training session. This was our warm-up.

Greg was the Vice President of a successful car company--most of you have owned at least one of his cars. Greg was white as a ghost; one of the only caucasian VP's in a predominantly Asian workplace. Greg spoke five languages well, and could hold his own with a few more. He traveled to places many folks will never go, and all well before he signed onto the biggest auto manufacturer in the world. For a white dude, he sure had some high-class Asians by the balls. He could deal with the Swedish, Spanish, American, and Asian divisions all on one conference call. Lets just say, Greg was in demand.

Luckily, for me anyway, Greg and I crossed paths as I began training his wife, who in her own right was a pocket genius like her husband. I think Greg simply gave into to his loving wife's nagging to come in for our first appointment. It was my personality, and our commonality, that kept Greg coming back. And no, I'm not intelligent, Greg's just generous. The only thing I had that he wanted was freedom … no stress for an hour.

Admittedly, Greg hated the training and since I adored my time learning from him, something I think he also enjoyed, I never really pushed him. We hit the bare minimum, and then chatted for as long as we could.

"Why?," Greg always asked with 12-year-old delight in his eyes. I loved that about him. Here was this VP of a billion dollar company asking me "why." The cool part was, he really listened to the answer.

By social standards and brain power, and just about everything else, Greg was light years ahead of me. Still, I was a break from the regular frazzled personalities Greg normally dealt with. I practiced a mindfulness that he needed to experience every so often. Like a surgeon who flies planes as a hobby, or a soldier who plays golf, he needed to take his mind off his duty.

Why Buddhist?
Buddhist's are pretty cool.

Real buddhists anyway, not the fake ones who mediate in the morning and get trashed at night. That's the same as christians who hate gay people.

Real buddhists tend to live long lives full of joy … and bad food.

How do they get away with it?

Mindfulness.

Mindfulness is the energy to be right here, right now, fully aware. Aware of everything happening within us and outside of us - present.

To be fully aware of each step, each bite, and each breath, means your mind isn't spinning. You're not preparing your argument waiting for your turn to talk, you're listening. You're not driving while making a to-do list, or texting. You're not walking while on a blue tooth preparing for a meeting eating a bagel. You're in the moment. The beautiful moment that has no stress.

I'm not a Buddhist, but I practice many of their techniques and some of the easiest that I learned from reading various Dhali's and monks may help you reach what I believe overcomes some of their nutritional nightmares: Mindfulness.

Breath

Monks practice various forms of meditation, some easier than others.

While I breath in, I will think "Calming," while I exhale I think, "Smiling." Inevitably, I smile. The very next segment of breath I think "present moment" while inhaling "Wonderful moment" while exhaling. Inevitably I smile.

This is simple when everything's going great, not so simple when everything sucks.

Anyone can smile while getting a tan but stepping back in the rain and making yourself breath and find joy is a critical personality trait that is so unnatural it must be practiced. It's like forgiveness; the reason we're commanded to forgive is because we wouldn't on our own. The reason it's difficult, and yet valuable, is because it's against our instincts. That's what makes it so special.

Walking

Tibetan Buddhists are so aware of nature that they won't leave their monastery during the rainy season. If they did, they take a chance of stepping on a worm. When is the last time you lived for something so small, so insignificant?

Whether you believe in karma or not, simply noticing how you treat a worm will echo loudly in how you treat a loved one.

When you walk, say "walking" over and over. The same goes with "sitting," "standing," "brushing," or whatever.

Repeat the words over and over in your mind when you approach these rather mindless activities and realize the beauty you have been missing when you walk your dog, do the dishes, or fold laundry. Beauty is everywhere and beauty is stressless.

Buddhist and Soy

A buddhist owns one bowl and two gowns. Or maybe it's the other way around, whatever. But you see I said bowl, not a knife or a fork. They don't need them to eat rice and soy. They're vegetarians.

Now, you can be a Paleo vegetarian, but I wouldn't recommend it. I also wouldn't recommend a very big part of an otherwise bland buddhist diet regime: Soy

Soy

The soybean originally came from Asia and was used as cheap livestock feed and packaging oi. Soy is served fermented and unfermented, and it's everywhere.

Fermentation aside - we can save that chat for another time - soy demonstrates many of the same dysfunctions all legumes while adding a few issues of its own. One or two make it particularly appealing to celibate monks.

Soy contains protease inhibitors. PH's are an allergen of sorts that make the enzymes required for nutrient breakdown and absorption stop.

Soy is an incomplete protein. Protein is essential Amino Acids that build and repair tissue. There are 21 amino acids depending on where you study. Out of those, ten are essential, meaning we must eat them because our body won't make them. While eating a variety of meat fulfills this requirement, eating soy does not.

Soy contains Phytates. Our "down to grains" chapter commented on this heavily but as a quick review; soy contains the same special grain antinutrient responsible for many many ailments plaguing us today. From CVD, Diabetes, Alzheimer's, Arthritis and more.

Soy gives you gas.
Soy has been linked to infertility. By spending your time eating tofu and carbohydrates while leaving meat in the freezer, you may shift your body into a strict survival mode conserving energy necessary for reproduction.

Soy increases estrogen and drops testosterone. Or maybe it drops testosterone and estrogen stays the same. Its doesn't matter. Testosterone makes you happy, lean, energetic. When you have virtually none, your a pissed off.

"Whether you believe in karma or not, simply noticing how you treat a worm will echo loudly in how you treat a loved one."

In fact, this one last point brings us back to Buddhists and their possible need for excessive meditation. Most Monks choose a life of celibacy. What better way to remain celibate than to eat something that makes your sex hormones shut off, then eliminate the female component so that life is automatically less stressful. Finally, mediate in Sangha's (virtuous communities) all day. Whala, instant stress free environment.

So I can't ever have Soy Sauce Again? What about the 80/20 rule?
Fitness guru's, fanatical diet practitioners and executive bigwigs love formulas and equations that can help define the undefinable--people. Pretty on paper is rarely beautiful when it counts--life.

In terms that my small mind can comprehend; the 80/20 rule (or Pareto Principle) states that for every event, 80% of the effect comes from 20% of the causes. For example, 80% of the countries wealth is controlled by 20% of the population, or 20% of farms grow 80% of the crops.

While I am by no means mathematically inclined enough to refute the numbers I often wonder why this measurement is even applied in the first place. After all, when are humans ever content with 80% of the results or only a portion of the blessings regardless of the work it takes to attain them?

Sometime ago the collective health and wellness experts with Four Hour Bodies and Paleo prescriptions began to apply this rule to food. Eating experts everywhere, including myself, concocted a means to the end WE wanted, not the one that was right. A Safari to keep pizza on the table is a trip worth skipping, not a bandwagon worth following.

While applying the 80/20 rule to your food and your ability to eat healthy "most of the time", you would tally up your meals through an entire week. For arguments sake, three meals a day, or twenty-one meals a week. By 80/20 standards, you would be more than welcome to consume four meals within that week that were very un-paleo. In fact, you were encouraged to "cheat".

"Fitness guru's, fanatical diet practitioners and executive bigwigs love formulas and equations that can help define the undefinable--people. Pretty on paper is rarely beautiful when it counts--life."

Promises of metabolism enhancement and thyroid stimulation clouded the literature in support of the cheat meal.

Manipulate the numbers long enough and your statistics will prove anything.

What if you twisted up that 80/20 principle and made it work against itself? How about, 20% of the poor food choices we make cause 80% of the problems, disease and disorders.

No, I may not fully believe that one pizza a week in the midst of Paleo living will cause a wealth of un-fixable issues. I may even go so far to say, other than multiple trips to the bathroom, that most of us would be no worse for wear. Except...

What if 20% of our actions create 80% of our addictions?

Harmlessly staring at a girl's butt on the street leads to cheating on your wife. One drink leads to AA, one pepperoni leads to owning a Domino's franchise. That's a big exception.

No savior would ever build an argument to allow atrocity. Saviors preach salvation at the cost of alienation. When applied to food, the 80/20 rule promotes addictions and prevents freedom.

It's fear. Fear is what bolsters a lifestyle lived below 100% dedication. Fear of failure. Our salvation is the knowledge that we were never guaranteed unending success anyway, we were granted the ability to be forgiven if we ask for it. The ability to triumph if we give our all, not some. Not 80%.

The 80/20 rule is a mathematical trick that is cool at bookkeeping parties and Paleo inspired t-shirts. It's not gospel, it's not healthy and it should not be recommended. Once we learn to aim small, we begin missing small. If your bulls-eye is 100%, near misses look a lot like direct hits.

Why I changed my mind
"When can we have you come down?," he asked, inviting me and my traveling seminar to his gym.

He wanted the best for the people he trained and when it comes to nutrition, he knew he wasn't the guy.

In two hours I spoke, we laughed, we issued a challenge and for weeks everyone got results. This is normal of course, but still very fun to watch and be a part of.

"Manipulate the numbers long enough and your statistics will prove anything."

Many athletes on the challenge started to blog their journey, many sent me question after question and I answered as fast as my hands would type. My friend had a great community and you could see it in their commitment to him and to the challenge.

Nearing the end of their 25-day-challenge, I got testimonials, pictures and all sorts of awesomeness I could share with the world. It was like a christmas of before and afters. Then the party came

"Come celebrate your victory," the email began. It ended with an address to a very un-paleo restaurant.

When you're addicted to bad food it takes longer than 30 days to get over it. The 30 day challenge is a bribe. Hopefully you feel so good you just keep going until the addiction lessens. Until finally, months and months later, it's gone. I think it took me seven months.

You see rewarding sobriety with beer only rewards Budweiser. For the person in recovery, they stop recovering.

Food is no different than alcohol. You would never take a recovering alcoholic out for a few beers after a month of sobriety, so why take fat people out for cake after a month paleo?

A few of my new friends even sent me pictures of deserts, hot wings and enormous pizza's. They were all smiles and their messages said something to the effect of, "look at our reward."

Luckily, I was far enough removed from the addiction that I could see it now. In fact, now I believe it takes that kinda person to really understand it. I was addicted all the same, but this time, nearly one year perfect paleo, I was cured and I knew what was coming - relapse.

"You would never take a recovering alcoholic out for a few beers after a month of sobriety, so why take fat people out for cake after a month paleo?"

The next day a couple people from their group emailed me and said they had food poisoning. They were right of course. Funny, there was nothing different about the food they ate that night than the food they used to eat one month prior. The difference is they were different.

In less than a month over half of athletes above had gained every single bit of their weight back. That's 20-30 lb. for some.

Their community of accountability had collapsed at the peak, my friend led the charge to get everyone on board and then he led the celebration to jump ship.

That was two years ago. Since then I have changed my prescription … 100% Paleo, 100% of the time.

Sober, after all, isn't just for alcoholics and Buddhists.

CHAPTER 7

WHY NOT THE FOOD PYRAMID, OR MY PLATE OR WHATEVER IT'S CALLED NOW

The plane left on time for once; Dayton to Chicago, and back to Dayton in the same day.

My job was to speak on "food and mood."

Usually I speak at schools, charitable events, round table discussions, so called expert panels and my own lectures. But this time it was for an up and coming company that looked like what I imagined Google to look like in it's infancy.

The company was owned by two young men, started in a basement. Both were about my age with absolutely no business background, just a passion for what they do. And man were they good at it.

My two entrepreneurial friends, Jason and Todd we'll call them, spent the bulk of their days arguing for the little guy ... guys like me. Guys like them.

Jason and Todd had passed the bar and were on their way to becoming successful litigators tackling everyday issues until a very dear friend of theirs lost his house, car, and everything he'd ever paid for. All because he signed something he didn't understand, and by the time they could do anything about it, it was too late. I'm sure you're guilty of this too ... ever click on the iTunes agree button without reading it?

My two lawyer buddies were motivated to start their now wildly successful practice that day because their friend signed a lease he shouldn't have. Todd and Jason reviewed their friends case and found many misleading, hidden and even quasi-illegal stipulations. Not only was the lease completely unjust, but so was the action taken when the lessee could not hold up to their end of the bargain.

From wrong came justice. Todd and Jason found their calling and their first client got his life back. They were so moved they took it upon themselves to fight for the little guy like a new age Robin Hood with a legal degree for a bow.

Even though it cost them everything

Ambulance chasers and divorce predators are just a few ways litigators capitalize on a dying world. If done correctly, it more than pays the bills. But fighting for the little guy, while blessed, doesn't exactly guarantee high society. Robin Hood, after all, lived in a tree.

Jason and Todd began fighting for those folks who needed help making their dreams come true when the powers that be were doing everything to make sure that didn't happen. At no charge they reviewed leases, argued terms and performed background checks. They worked out of their basement nearly starving until a rather wealthy well connected individual heard of their exploits. The law firm this gentleman owned was so impressed that they were willing to finance some of their work, assuming they could get credit for it in the press.

Thankfully, this wasn't the only reward. J&T quickly became its own charity, raising funds for "the little guy." Sort of a community RRG (Risk Retention Group) in the ghetto.

I met them by doing what I love; CrossFit. The affiliate they trained at, asked if I'd come and chat about food.

About 18 months earlier, J&T witnessed one of my speeches and was impressed enough to hang out afterwards. The three of us were fast friends and have remained in touch to this day.

Long after J&T and I met they continued the CrossFit+Paleo adventure. But like most of us, they noticed that no matter the example they set, others just didn't follow.

Sure, they'd taken a few people to workout and like anything else, go to church long enough and you're gonna start believing. But the overwhelming majority of their now powerful organization were still sick and in need, living a drive-thru lifestyle.

The Set-up

"Josh, can you give a motivational seminar to our employees?," Jason asked.

"You know I don't do that," I said. "People may become motivated, but I'm no Tony Robbins."

"Yeah yeah, when can you come,?" Jason asked.

I stopped arguing after I remembered that I was talking to a lawyer.

The worst seminars are the ones where I know people don't want to change. The ones where someone invited me as an icebreaker to a conversation everyone hates. It makes me sweat just thinking about the roomful of forlorn glances and ready death-threats. I've been scolded at churches, shunned at schools and banished from entire cities ... it feels like it anyway.

What made this speech so noteworthy was that it would be given to over 60 lawyers, paralegals and their assistants. People that argued for a living. Not only that, but these people didn't want to change. They were prepared to argue for their way of life.

How do you make a room full of vipers change their minds?

First, you don't call them vipers, they're people and they want to feel good. Jason and Todd knew this, and they couldn't, in good conscious, let their friends die of disease.

Population Control

Most folks would say that there is no way our government would have been feeding us nutritional lies for the past century. But then again, who says they did it knowingly. A conspiracy can start honestly and it usually does. Good intentions get confused with too much pride and no-one wants to admit that they're the cause for a dying nation.

I'm unsure if I believe the government's goal with the Lipid Hypothesis was holocaust by nutrition, or just outright ignorance. In truth, it doesn't matter what the intention was when we recommend a low fat/high carb diet decades ago. What matters is that it's killing us today.

In the 20s we never had heart attacks or cancers to speak of. By the 50's we did. And the worse it got the louder the outcry. The louder the demand to answer the pressing questions, "why are we sick?"

Years after the low fat/high carb become the food messiah, critics started watching numbers. Everything got worse, and there was no way to deny it.

The Basic Four

Even before the discovery of vitamins and minerals our nation was recognizing the importance of food. Guidelines were established as early as the 1900s.

Ever changing as those guidelines may have been, they originally had merit. It was the definition that failed.

In the forties we didn't have the food pyramid. We had "The Basic Four:" Meat, milk, fruit and vegetables. Even though I dislike the milk thing, you can imagine how much better off we would be if we forever left it at the basics.

But just because it didn't make the list of the Basic Four doesn't mean it wasn't produced.

Agricultural companies began to flood the market with cereal grains and shelved items that held longer and tasted better. The nation ignored the basic four, and forced the government to live up to the wrongful definition of the food pyramid, the definition that is killing us today.

Food Pyramid Credo: Moderation/Proportionality/Variety:
Those administering the guidelines that would soon become Egyptian mob rule, added a fifth group to the basic four by the 70's, giving people the luxury to eat grains and sweets. Not because we should, because we demanded it, and because their definition forces it.

They came up with a slogan unhealthy Americans sing until their deathbeds. "Everything in moderation."

Moderation
There is no other species as bright and as blessed as us. We are creators. Thinkers. Images of something greater than we can imagine.

From us comes advancement and progress thought impossible just decades ago. But with that comes the scariest form of corruption we face today... technology.

Not because technology in itself is bad. No, we are truly better off than our Paleolithic ancestors. When they sprained an ankle they were left for dead. When they couldn't catch a fish they starved. When they got a scrape, they got infected. No, our technology is our gift to ourselves, but with it comes with one universal requirement most of us forget to apply for our entire lives: discipline.

We spend so much time arguing about how to do something, we forget to ask if we should. It is awesome we can keep sugar filled snack cakes from spoiling while on the shelves for years, but does that make it right?

No, creating things in a lab and calling it "additive" or "other ingredients" is not a blessing. It's our curse of technology running wild because we have no discipline in application. There is no room for moderation in a world of blurred boundaries.

Variety
Variety is spoon-fed to us everyday. We believe we need it, and by all means, we deserve it.

Variety in marriage is called adultery. Variety in religion is called damnation. It's not that it can't be used for good, it's that today, variety is an excuse. Variety is defensive and keeps up from commitment.

Our ancestors did not have the cereal aisle. Or any other aisle for that matter.

Their utter lack of variety is what kept them alive and un-addicted. Food was believed to be, and still should be, nothing more than energy. When we make it an event, when we think we're deserving of new and special recipes and sources, we get bored. When we get bored, we eat.

If you only were allowed to eat once a day, wouldn't you appreciate your food more? Wouldn't anything be better than nothing? Wouldn't plain chicken always taste great?

Today, however, we have abundance. We recommend eating three to five meals a day. We constantly have a new version of the same old thing simply because we keep that definition alive. The definition that says variety is essential to life, when more often than not, it's the exact opposite.

Proportionate

"Control your portions and you will lose weight" is what companies like Weight Watchers spread throughout the land. All evidence to the contrary, of course.

Sure, reducing your Calories may, most likely for a short lived time, reduce your weight on the scale. But it won't change your waist size or reflection much.

Poor food choices, even at "better proportions" still lead to poor results. Skinny fat is a term you hear thrown around today. It means you still take up the same amount of room in this world, you're just fatter and with less muscle.

In the truest sense, we cannot have our cake and eat it too. Alcoholics don't get "portion control." They get "cold turkey."

Lawyers, treatment, and the vicious cycle

As I wrapped up my seminar to the poker faces in front of me I said this;

"You're part of a global conspiracy to prescribe a method of drug intervention called diet. This so called diet gives way to various behaviors, addictions, and eventually afflictions that will require another prescription just to maintain degrading health. But not so degrading you'll die, just harmful enough to need another prescription. This vicious cycle will continue, unabated, and even celebrated, as an example of our infinite intelligence and progress as a society. Not only will this prescription keep you funding your own demise, it will make the bars of your cage stronger, until one day you're too sick and tired to care that you're in prison at all."

I rest my case....

CHAPTER 8

WHY DO I FEEL LIKE CRAP?

When my phone rings and it says "blocked" I ignore it.

It makes me think of the movie Scream where the guy called everyone before he chopped them up. Luckily, at least for Tom, I answered.

"Josh?," he asked before I said hello. "Yup," I said. "This is Tom, Maggie's husband, you got a minute?," he asked.

I had never talked to, or met, Tom. I worked for his wife. But the moment he got that sentence out, I knew where this was going. Maggie was on her first contest diet, and she was entering Ketosis. She hadn't had carbs for a week. Poor Tom was the guy living with her.

"Sure thing Tom, everything ok; Maggie seem more like a stranger and less than your wife these days?," I asked pre-empting the storm. The phone went silent for a second. I could hear the edgy pissed off in Tom's voice when he finally responded."

"Yeah, how did you know?"

"Well Tom, I trained her this morning, and it's not just you she is giving the cold shoulder to. And before we go on, It ain't your fault, it's mine."

Tom immediately settled down like a kid learning the reason for their parents divorce wasn't because he didn't clean his room. Tom believed Maggie was upset with him. He had never witnessed this "different" version of her. The poor guy's mind was running wild all week.

In a world where we get divorced because our significant other forgot the cream in our coffee, where even the smallest voice inflections are taken out of context and turned into carnal sins, a wife with no carbs is an A-bomb.

"Tom, did Maggie tell you I changed her diet this week?," I asked.

"Yeah."

"Well, do you know what that means? I took away her carbs, Tom."

"So, what's that mean; and if you took them, why is she punishing me?"

Huh, a logical come back I hadn't expected. This whole mess was common back when I began prescribing diets. I was a rookie following experienced teachers who had the mechanics wrong. I paid the price for following instead of thinking.

Maggie was uncomfortable because I was dieting her the way trainers had dieted me. The suffer way not the success way.

We've watched Rocky IV too many times. What else could explain the notion that health must hurt and that athletics must be difficult to work. Now, I'm not saying that it isn't intense, and that you won't have to lay it down, but I still think it can be mostly fun, and rewarding. It doesn't have to suck to work, or to be worth it.

"In a world where we get divorced because our significant other forgot the cream in our coffee, where even the smallest voice inflections are taken out of context and turned into carnal sins, a wife with no carbs is an A-bomb."

I finally realized that after my second bodybuilding show. I was fed up with treating my brother like crap, driving by Burger King just to smell awesome, and feeling like my legs were glued to the floor.

Sadly, at least for Tom and Maggie, this revelation came long after her competitive career had ended. But hey, Tom, and Maggie still have a laugh or two about those unforgettable few weeks without carbs, the old-school way.

Well, Maggie laughs more than Tom.

Old School

The way it was, and still is for much of the population, is off-season and in-season. Supposedly they compliment each other, They made me insane.

It reminds me of a convertible in the summer. You gas it up with top notch fuel, you wash and wax it constantly, you even drive it just to see what it's capable of, not just to go somewhere. Then, when the summers over, you leave is rotting beneath two feet of snow all winter.

"We're dying one luxury at a time."

Healthy has no offseason.

Old school says take a healthy timeout, eat whatever, and then when you want to be healthy again, it's gonna hurt. Well I'm here to tell you that I can cure the food addiction that even makes this seem reasonable, and that it doesn't hurt at all.

Welcome to new school fitness where everyday is a healthy day.

Ketosis 101

Ketosis is a normal and healthy state for humans to live in. In fact, many organs prefer ketosis, including your heart.

When you can "shift" your body, or induce keto-adaptation, you change it's energy source to ketones - think fat, think cholesterol and triglycerides.

The biggest difference between cholesterol and triglycerides is that cholesterol isn't going to be released as energy, it's going to enhance cell integrity, serve as an antioxidant and anti-psychotic, repair arterial walls, enhance immune function, improve cognitive resonance and ensure the proper hormone chain is effective when producing things like testosterone, vitamin-D, and prostaglandins.

Triglycerides, on the other hand, can be broken down into the more basic glycerol molecule, and three chain fatty acid. This is how someone on low carb diet can have a high fasting blood glucose by the way. This is why FBG is paired with an H1ac test to ensure accuracy.

Ketosis keeps glucagon high, which releases energy through fat. Therefore, insulin is incredibly low because insulin stores fat instead of burns it. Reaching the "shift" eliminates energy peaks and valleys, stops many cancers and diseases, and crushes food and alcohol addiction.

And don't get this confused with ketoacidosis - where the body cannot utilize glucose properly due to diabetes and the individual breaks down fats, overwhelming the body with acid. This is fatal if left untreated, but it only happens to diabetics to my knowledge. The telltale signs are; really fruity or blood breath, nausea, nasty smelling pee and sweat...you would know.

Our ancestors were ketotic

High blood pressure, type II diabetes, obesity, and several other disease exist because we don't live for the season.

T.S Wiley authored an astounding read "Lights Out, Sleep, Sugar, Survival", I recommended it. To summarize; Wiley says we're animals. Like bears in the summertime, we get fat. Carbohydrates are abundant so we eat them, then we get lazy have lots of sex and party like a rock star with the extended daylight hours.

We become hypertensive to conserve sodium. We also develop insulin resistance and carry about 20 lb. of excess water, all natural and healthy occurrences under the right circumstances. But here is the thing, we would only be like this for the short summer months. The rest of the time we would be surviving on fats and meat, no green or carbs to speak of.

Basically, summertime would prime the pump for a naturally ketotic, and healthy, winter. We would burn all that stored fat as ketones for fuel, and we would transform from fat to fit over the course of a few cold months.

Think of ketosis as a garbage disposal. You can pile it up and leave it for the next day, or the day after that. Either way it still works, but everybody just makes it stink a little more. Ketosis is nature's way of cleaning up the excessive side of humans, the addictive side.

The Ketosis Cure

Dr. Warburg, way back into the the 1920s', discovered what could arguably be called the cure for cancer. "Starvation."

Cancer cells are present in all of us. For instance BRCA 1 and 2, found in women who suffer from breast cancer, is also found in women who don't. We are born with these so called "bad" genes. Its called "genotyping". But born with, in most cases, doesn't mean live with. That's called phenotyping, and that's how we express our genes.

Dr. Warburg figured out that cancer usually eats sugar, and that if you feed the body tons of fat, it basically starves to death. He was even awarded the Nobel Prize for this discovery. But of course, shortly after his discovery, some other guys discovered cancer treatment was far more profitable than a cancer cure.

Epilepsy

Proven not only effective, but crucial for epileptics, ketosis eliminates anywhere from 40 - 100 percent of seizures, depending on the patient. And when it comes to kids, the statistics get better.

It's not even proven how ketosis truly works to diminish or halt seizures all together, but who really cares what goes in the black box if what comes out is so helpful.

Humans are a series of electrical impulses. That's why electrolytes are so critical. Unfortunately, some are born with a constant electrical storm going on. Glucose makes the storm worse and the body adapts to a sugar metabolism. But adaptation doesn't mean preferential and just because it works doesn't make it right. Ketones are actually the body's preferred source of fuel.

The goal is to rid the body of abundance. Too much glucose, too many Calories, too much whatever and you have your recipe for a dish you won't enjoy. This is why the bible says, "give us this day our daily bread." To me, that means just enough, never too much.

We're dying one luxury at a time.

I know this is ultra simple, but can't epileptics just be very poor at utilizing glucose, can't epilepsy be diabetes IV, just as Alzheimer's is diabetes III?

Alzheimer's and other neurodegenerative disorders

Diabetes is really glucose poisoning. The different versions - I and II - refer to born with, or created. Two is self-inflicted resistance to insulin built over time. One is the disorder we are born with where our pancreas does not release the proper hormone amount at the right time. Either way, glucose is the issue. Prolonged exposure to glucose over the years wears out certain parts of the brain making memory, and other neurological functions impossible.

" … who really cares what goes in the black box if what comes out is so helpful."

Alzheimers, also called diabetes III, is prolonged exposure to glucose. We poison ourselves with sugar until we can't remember who we are.

How To "Shift"

The "Shift" refers to Keto-adaptation or becoming efficient at burning ketones for fuel as opposed to glucose. Just like anything else, the first couple times usually sucks, but the more you do it the better you get. Thankfully we have my many mistakes to guide us down the much simpler, and faster, path to ketotic greatness.

Ketotic In 6 Steps...

1. Eliminate all carbs now (except greens). Carboholics are the same as alcoholics. You don't tell alcoholics to have nine beers tomorrow, then eight next week. You send alcoholics to detox and let them suffer withdrawal. Without withdrawal there is no cure.

    When Alcoholics leave the sauce behind most fill the void with sugar. That's what they really enjoyed about the alcohol anyway. Remember alcohol bypasses the stomach and essentially becomes one of the fastest sugar delivery methods there is. Why do you think AA meetings are full of doughnuts, coffee and nicotine?

2. Start taking 20-grams of glutamine per day.

    Glutamine is a glycogenic amino acid that can kill carb and alcohol cravings. When in the presence of zero carbs the brain will recognize glutamine as sort of the fog lifter during the "shift" period. Some of us don't need this, some do.

    Each week after you begin taking glutamine, remove five grams from your dose.

3. When we say eliminate carbs I mean heavy starchy carbs, and admittedly any carb amounting to much of anything other than trace amounts.

Some of us reach ketosis at just under 100 g/day, some 50 g/day, some less. You're going to have to play with it for a bit, but eventually you will hit your sweet spot.

Most carb sources should be the carbs from nuts and green vegetables.

4. Drink water. Ketones must be processed and if we are poorly hydrated they will come out in our breath. If you notice a fruity odor in your breath, you're not drinking enough. I would start at ½ body-weight in ounces a day, and raise from there.

5. Start 2,000 mg of L-Carnitine/day. LC acts like an amnio but it's not. LC helps shuttle fat into the mitochondria more efficiently. Glutamine halts cravings, LC burns fat better.

6. If you're not already, begin taking MCT (medium-chain-triglyceride) oil. Coconut oil is 75% MCT. MCT's, among other things, promote the burning of ketones more than any other nutrient. MCT's also allow slightly more carbohydrates to be present while still maintaining ketosis.

Maggie and Tom

Recently I had dinner with Maggie and Tom. Maggie I see all the time, but not Tom. He doesn't workout and he travels a lot. I almost didn't recognize him.

"What happened, you get sick?," I said like a prick.

Tom hated dieting. Especially after Maggie nearly divorced him during her first show.

"Sick of being fat," he said.

By the time the bland pleasantries were over the waitress was hovering over our table. We all ordered steak, except me of course, I got steak and ribs.

"So what changed, Tom?," I asked. I figured the doctor showed him something that scared him. Or maybe he was playing with one of his kids and passed out. You would be surprised how often I hear that.

"You made eating easy," he said. "When I saw Maggie eating most of the things I liked, and still looking the way she wanted, I figured why not. That was nine months ago."

Tom said he lost 32 lb. eating steak for dinner every night. Sometimes he ate salads for appetizers.

"Oh," Tom said smiling, "and I never had to do that crazy stuff you guys do either."

I still do my best to make Tom a CrossFitter, but in the meantime, at least he's getting the most out of his food. At least it's not killing him anymore.

CHAPTER 9

STOP EATING BREAKFAST

When I was growing up, my mom worked from dark to dark. Dad was gone and we had to eat.

She dropped me off at school, kissed my cheek under protest, and drove to one of the many clothing stores she managed. Six days a week, well past TV's prime time, I heard the garage open and ran to the door, excited to see my mom, tired of being alone and hungry for the bag of food she'd always bring.

I love my mom very much.

As a kid I never ate before the afternoon. In the morning I slept until the two minute warning, then put pants and a shirt on before running out the door just in time to be 5-minutes late everywhere. At lunch I saved my money so I could buy candy with my friends on the walk home.

For years, all the way through my high school career in fact, I never ate before 3 p.m. But from three-o'clock on, it was like an eating contest that I always won.

Twizzlers, Snickers and Mountain Dew were appetizers. When I got home I microwaved something that looked and smelled like pizza, then rushed back to my friends until I got hungry again. After mom and I shared our brown bag dinner, I had dessert; Lucky Charms.

That was everyday for me for a very long time. That's everyday for a lot of us.

My 18-year-old birthday present to myself was a gym membership. My first legal contract motivated from years of GI-Joe cartoons, and violent movies. I'd always wanted to look like a superhero and I couldn't recall too many 140 lb. Batman renditions.

I gained weight.

Break The Fast forever:
The media driven diet dogma we're all taught to believe says; "eat a huge breakfast, it's the most important meal of the day. Breakfast gets the metabolism revved up so you can burn fat. It provides energy".

These are all statements we have heard and worshipped. And they're wrong, created by Jimmy Dean, Bob Evans, Met-RX, Taco-bell, Kroger and anyone else who can profit from you eating more food, more often.

Today there's enough food processed in America for humans to consume 4000/cal day. Coincidentally, there is 12+ billion dollars in advertising spent per year to make you buy your 4000/cal.

If I skip Breakfast; won't I get Fat?
Years ago I would have said, yes.

Back then, even though I knew better like many of us, I would blindly follow supplement companies, and commercials, and cute little magazines all preaching the same thing; eat early, eat often, stoke the fire.

I would simply avoid the most basic law of thermodynamics applied to the human body. Calories in vs Calories out. You will get fat if you eat too many of the wrong Calories. You will lose weight if you burn more than you take in.

Remember insulin, the storage hormone? Insulin ensures we keep fat (energy) on us for times of famine. Clearly, with 4000 Calories a day, we won't starve anytime soon.

Blood glucose is generally at it's lowest point in the morning when we have went without eating for some time. Biology 101 says to stay fasted as long as possible. Keep insulin levels low because once they rise we can't burn fat for energy. In essence, when you wake-up, you're burning fat for fuel, after you eat your burning off food. Stay fit, stay fasted.

If I don't eat Breakfast, won't I have less energy?
After much experimentation on myself and others, and remembering finally what I was taught in school, not in the funny pages, the answer is a loud, "NO".

In fact, you'll have so much more energy you won't know what to do with yourself and you'll annoy everyone around you.

When you rise in the morning cortisol is high and insulin is low, You were designed to be active, to kill, hunt, survive. Your Sympathetic Nervous System (SNS) or fight or flight is turned on. We are taught cortisol is our stressful killer and we need to keep it at bay at all times. Per usual, it's not that simple. Truth is, we need to pay more attention to keeping cortisol balanced like our ancestors did.

Remaining driven by your natural SNS in the morning utilizes fat for fuel, provides mounds of energy and does everything but allow us to tire out. Eating immediately kicks the antagonistic PSNS in, which regulates digestion and relaxation. Hardly the way we want to attack the day.

Adding insult, or insulin rather, to injury we are taught to carb the crap out of breakfast. Hmmmmm … eating a ton of carbs early simply ensures we experience reactive hypoglycemia a couple hours later and feel like we'll die unless we eat again.

Eating Breakfast doesn't give you energy, it stops energy, makes you lethargic and ensures you buy more to eat in few hours.

Ok … but what If I work out in the morning, should I eat before?
Take full advantage of your fat burning capabilities and workout fasted. Suck it up at first, it will get better.

Training fasted is one of the quickest ways to fat loss you can imagine. When we are fasted there is no insulin or calories hanging out blunting our fat burning. Nor is there a relaxed state to overcome because you're already ramped up. Simply make your post workout meal(most important meal of the day) your first meal of the day.

Won't I Lose Muscle?
No.

Muscle gain is directly related to protein intake, consistency, and exercise. Blast away at yourself time and time again and in short bouts. Eat at least .5 to .75 grams of protein per pound of body-weight, and make sure you define protein as something that roamed the earth at one time or another. In fact, remaining in a fasted state will actually preserve muscle, and teach the body to better utilize fat burning.

Are you Jackin' with me, is there anything else I need to know before I give up the "most important meal of the day?"
Nope.

Caffeine is fine and may even enhance the effects. As far as other supplements, L-Glutamine helps fight cravings and L-Carnitine helps the mitochondria use fat more efficiently.

Also, carb burners who have yet to adopt a low carb intake enough to promote ketosis may find skipping BF uncomfortable at first ... good. This too shall pass.

Lastly, don't be that guy who gives a million reasons why you're different than every other human and, "this just can't work because you need your morning oats," speech. Step out of your comfort zone and put down your morning bagel for a big glass of try something new.

CHAPTER 10

WHY FAT

"My strength lies in my asking people to do nothing that I have not tried repeatedly in my own life"

-Ghandi

"Can you tell me how the diets going Jimmy?," my dad's doctor asked.

My dad was overweight - imagine John Candy - diabetic and a stroke victim. When someone made him nervous he stuttered like a typewriter missing a key.

"Go .. go...good," my Dad said smiling like a toddler getting ready to poke you with something sharp.

"You're not doing what I asked are you."

"Well, some of it."

"Oh yeah, Jimmy," the doctor said.

I feel for the guy. His average patient is waiting to die and wants to get to the grave as pain free as possible. That was my dad. That's America.

Still talking to my dad like a principal talks to a 12-year-old who just got caught smoking, the doc says, "which part are you doing?"

"I'm eating more fruit."

Conveniently, I missed our last appointment where the doctor had slipped in the diet talk without me. At least in my hometown I'm popular enough that everybody knows what I do and many know what I believe. The only reason I keep trekking my father back is because old folks fear change like kids fear needles.

"What did you tell him to change?," I asked.

"Nothing drastic. Eat more fruit and veggies, drink low-fat milk, eat lots of whole grains to replace the candy and give up all that saturated fat. I didn't try to take away his food, I just want him to make better choices."

"I didn't try to take away his food, I just want him to make better choices."

- Dr.

It felt like I was on an elevator and my stomach felt the shift in altitude. I finally understood what the guy holding the stethoscope was trying to do. For the first time since I thought I had all the answers, I wanted to help.

The doctor and I had the same goals, but one of us had the wrong info. Gandhi says, "We are all liable to err. But it is our duty to correct our errs."

Even so, health professionals can only give cures patients are willing to follow. Pills, after all, are a lot lighter than barbells, and a lot more fun than running.

My dad took part of his doctors advice. Not surprisingly, the part about adding sugar. His fat content, as you would have guessed, stayed the same.

A little fatty flavor
Fat is good for you.

I don't think I have to say much more … it just is.

It was Ancel Keys who started the whole vilify fat and celebrate carbo-hydrate thing back in the fifties. If you want to know the story google it. It's been disproven by everyone.

The reason we still follow his recommendation 50-years in the future is the scary thing.

Kwik E Marts + Oil=Metabolic Syndrome
AC started the trouble when he said reduce fat, blaming cholesterol for the nation's demise. We know now that reducing cholesterol intake promotes more cholesterol production. We also know if you reduce your Caloric intake from fat, you make up the reduction with carbohydrates. And once carbohy-drates are the main source of Calories, insulin runs rampant only to combine with the uptake of serum cholesterol now being produced. Whala...CVD, Metabolic Syndrome, Stroke, Death.

"Even so, health professionals can only give cures patients are will-ing to follow. Pills, after all, are a lot lighter than barbells, and a lot more fun than running."

To say sugar is addictive is to say the sun is hot. We know it is, and we all love it. Lazy is also addictive and lots of us love that too. Keys gave us the coffin in the fifties. The nail came in the 80's with the invention of the convenience store

Think of it like a three step process. First, sell a lie that makes a lot of money=coffin. Second, have the ability to sell the lie 24-hours-a-day-seven-days-a-week=nails. Third, put gas pumps in front=dirt.

In 2009 the convenience store industry posted annual sales of 511 billion dollars. Just over half of that was gas.

When the first "Kwik E Mart" opened back in the 80's it only offered Twinkie's, Slushies and Pepsi. America was Alice getting her first glimpse of the white rabbit. When they decided to keep their doors open 24/7/365, we decided to show up a little more often to thank them.

Exxon and BP eventually discovered that Americans could set the pump to fill while buying a treat to hold them over for the long trip to the nearest drive-thru.

Keys, the government, school lunches get the bad press for a nation of big bellies, but it's not their fault. Our epidemic of fat is based off our obsession for convenience.

Gas+sugar=antichrist.

Keys did one bad study and Big Soda and everyone else who stood to gain from his shady science jumped on the attack fat bandwagon.

Because sugar is addictive, and convenience is, well, convenient, we kept believing him even when the feedback was diabetes, heart disease and death. You can't place the blame on him any more than you can the head of BP.

And for that matter, who can blame Pfizer, or Merck for making drugs that are easier to take than exercise. Drugs that simply prolong our ability to buy more drugs, fill more gas tanks and drink more Squishes.

The Real World

When MTV put a camera in a house full of idiots and called it prime time bad went to worse.

Now reality is on TV and life is the illusion. A confession booth where grown men talk about their feelings is plastered all over the airwaves for other adolescent males to see.

Generations grow up talking not doing.

"To say sugar is addictive is to say the sun is hot. We know it is, and we all love it. Lazy is also addictive and lots of us love that too."

Before I go on let me make a qualification. I'm not horribly sexist. I believe women and men are equal. But I believe women are easily better at certain things than men. Just as men are better at so called manly things.

I believe in a certain kind of primordial behavior we would all do well to adhere to. No, I'm not going to club the next pair of long legs strolling by and drag her home. But if someone treated her poorly in front of me it would be my duty to stand up for her honor. Just because some women feel oppressed by stereotypes doesn't mean they're not true, it means some women are too sensitive.

Men are supposed to lead and leaders can't lead by emotion. All the Real World reality show did was add emotion to the emotionless. There are just things that don't matter, but all of the sudden dudes bitched about daddy working too much, or hitting the bottle every night, or never saying "I love you."

It started with Apu running the little shop on the corner, it got worse when the shop got gas, it became chronic when we added emotion. Once something goes chronic it can finally be treated, not cured. Pfizer created numbers to live by. Numbers like cholesterol, triglycerides, blood pressure. Then we bought their drugs to keep us in line with "their" numbers.

If you're a man, shut up.

Walk through a field with a gun, kill something, grill it and eat. Drive something that makes sense, but do it less often than others, learn to walk more and sprint some. Stop going to the mall or Home Depot. Drive to the mountains to camp and to a gym to WOD, to a diamond to watch your kids play ball. Watch a movie on Saturdays and most importantly, Confess to God, not a camera in a booth.

Panopticon

Jeremy Bentham created a prison where one guard could watch hundreds of prisoners by eliminating the population's ability to see their captor. His prison was ruled by the fear of what if. "What if I am being watched?"

Simply extend Bentham's idea. Cameras on every corner a chip in every palm, a GPS on every human. Tagged and bagged before we take our last breath. At least convicts see the bars surrounding them.

"When MTV put a camera in a house full of idiots and called it prime time bad went to worse."

Maybe the powers that be found something better than a camera on every corner and fear in every heart. Maybe our prison is plaque in every artery and medication in every cabinet.

"All hail Pfizer."

"Thanks be to Hostess."

We were led into our cage by way of old fashioned propaganda for the two oldest reasons in the book. Money and control. Those at the top want to keep the top so badly they find a way to drug those on the bottom. Just enough to keep us docile slow and scared. Those at the bottom are too scared to lose their cupcakes. To freighted to miss a dose.

Bentham's modern day panopticon is carbohydrates. Pharmacists are the guards.

Fatty variety:
When compared to our supposedly preferred fuel - glucose - fat delivers a knockout punch every time. We have about enough glucose stored as glycogen in our liver and muscles to last us a day. Even an ultra lean Ab queen has enough body fat to last a month. Fat offers nine Calories of energy per gram versus carbohydrates four calories.

Fat forms almost all brain and nerve matter. Fat, via cholesterol, is like the bodies sewer crew keeping the pipes clean and in working order. Limiting fat is limiting maintenance. And the older you get, the more essential proper maintenance becomes.

Fats are generally categorized by the carbon chain trailing them; long, medium or short. They're either Saturated, Monounsaturated or Polyunsaturated.

For instance Coconut oil, a Saturated Fat, contains medium chain triglycerides. Meaning, it bypasses much of the lymphatic system where most fats are lead, and it is absorbed much faster into the bloodstream like carbohydrates. All without the insulin spike of carbs. The body then will burn this as fuel along with other body fat, unless you eat carbs, then it just burns that.

Fats contain carbon, oxygen, and hydrogen. A saturated fat is simply full of hydrogen at every location possible, and every carbon atom single bonded. Therefore making a carbon chain with only one double bond of carbon Monounsaturated, and polyunsaturated being multiple double bonds present within the fatty chain.

"Just because some women feel oppressed by stereotypes doesn't mean they're not true, it means some women are too sensitive."

Saturated has no double bonds of carbon, and unsaturated has the affinity for one double bond or more. For instance, a polyunsaturated with a double bond starting at the third carbon atom form the methyl end or n-3 end would be Omega 3. Trans fats are there too … but we will hit that later.

One of the biggest differences is the more double bonds a fat contains the quicker it usually oxidizes or breakdown to give off its energy. The quicker something oxidizes, the quicker it becomes rancid. Some fats are so quick to become rancid that just leaving them on the counter starts fires, others can be exposed to air for years and be fine.

Fats are really meant to be called lipids as "fats" means solid at room temperature, and oils are well oils. Generally, saturated fat is more solid at room temperature. Think butter and coconut oil. Unsaturated fats are more liquid like olive oil and the like.

Fat is an essential nutrient like protein, unlike carbohydrates. Meaning the body cannot produce them so we must get them through our diet. In other words crucial to live. They are essential for many of the reasons listed above, but also for vitamin absorption. Ever heard of fat soluble vitamins? Yup it's like it sounds, without dietary fat, you can't absorb vitamins A, D, E, and K.

Last but not least, and covered a few chapters over. Fat satisfies Leptin, the master hunger hormone telling you when you're full. Eating fat makes you full, if you're full, you're not eating, if you're not eating, it's harder to get fat.

Triglyceride
Once fat enter the body they begin the whole pretty digestive process of 453 steps or so. Lipase begins to break it down as well as the bile produced from the gall bladder (hint hint, you need your gallbladder, God didn't mess up).

The bile produced by the liver and stored in the GB emulsifies fat so that the digestive enzymes can do their jobs. After all, oil and water don't mix. The bile salts do their job allowing the water soluble lipase to finally have a go at digesting the fat. Bile ensures almost all fat we eat is digested. Without bile you can hardly digest even nominal amounts of fat. You ever wonder why folks that have had their gallbladder removed can't eat fat?

Depending on the fat eaten of course (short and medium chain are absorbed straight to the bloodstream like alcohol and don't need the lymphatic system) you're ready to roll with the most energizing source of food we have. Maybe the best nutrient available besides air and water.

Eventually you have triglycerides or a three chain fatty acid with a glycerol backbone. Used correctly, this is the best source of energy a human can have. The main difference between triglycerides and cholesterol is triglycerides are burned for energy assuming no energy substrates like carbs get in the way.

The reason why your triglycerides are high isn't because you eat a lot of fat, it's because you eat carbs and your body isn't good at burning fat. If you wanna be good at something do it often.

Eating fat makes your body really good at burning fat. Triglycerides are not a measure of fat in the blood, they are a measure of carbs eaten, and therefore insulin secreted.

Specifically Saturated:
As I mentioned above, saturated fats are more tightly packed, usually appear solid at room temperature, and have a longer life that of unsaturated fats. I could go on, but instead I would refer you to "Know Your Fats", by Mary Enig PHD. This 400 page tome can describe everything I am leaving out.

"The idea that saturated fat causes heart disease is completely wrong, but the statement has been published so many times over the past three or more decades that it

*is very difficult to convince people otherwise unless they are willing to take the time
to read and learn what produced the anti-saturated fat agenda."*

-Mary Enig

Saturated fat has become the scapegoat for every case of CVD in the country. As stated above, SF sources include Coconut, Butter, Cream, Eggs, Meat.

SF Benefits:
Your heart muscle works better.

Saturated fat raises HDL (high density lipids-good cholesterol).

Cell walls become stronger. When trans fat are gone, and carbs aren't the main course, cells use fat as glue for repair

Improve gut health, stimulate gut fighting bacteria. Specifically MCT. These little wonders ward off offending agents due to the Lauric acid and other compounds that are inert to us, but hell to our enemies.

Drastically improve bone health. Calcium is great for bones also, but only if it's absorbed. When we ensue 50-percent of our total fat is saturated, we create an environment primed to soak up calcium.

Improves Omega 3 absorption. Omega 3 is a polyunsaturated fat, but without its brother, saturated fat, it cannot bring the party to the party goers.

Makes you lean. The more fat you eat, the less carbs, the more full you feel, and the better you become at burning fat.

Monounsaturated fat:
Saturated fat has all single bonds of carbon because carbon is one of the few elements that forms rings of atoms joined by chemical bonds in which, one, two or three electrons can be paired. MUFA's have one double bond of carbon.

Think olive oils, avocados, some nuts, and even meat has some MUFAs.

I'm not fond of using olive oil for cooking in the least, it has a lower smoke point than saturated fats, meaning it oxidizes quickly because it isn't as tightly packed chemically. Basically MUFA go rancid faster. However, when you can find it, avocado oil has the highest smoke point of any oil rolling in at 510 degrees, making it better than coconut.

MUFA's Benefits:

Improved insulin sensitivity. When we have less insulin wafting through our bloodstream, we remember more, live longer, age gracefully and look leaner. We have less insulin because in a healthy body, a little goes a long way. Remember insulin stores stuff (fat), glucagon releases stuff (fat or energy from fat).

Heavy antioxidant content. It's impossible to exclude all known carcinogens from our diet. Hell sleeping with a night light on is a carcinogen. But antioxidants act as armor to the inevitable.

Decreased cholesterol. MUFA's seem to lower total cholesterol count. But like we mentioned, this is kinda "eh".

Polyunsaturated Fatty Acids:

Arguably the most widely used fat source on the market today, PUFA are found in just about everything. From baked goods to wild caught fish, and they come with a host of issues.

PUFA's are harmful because we're not prepared to handle how they come at us. Take the Omega's for instance - 3 and 6. Both are PUFA's and both are essential, meaning your body can't make them so you must eat them to live. Nature had a plan to give us a certain ratio, we simply changed the plan. Omega 6 is cheaper, so we get far more of. It's like rain, enough makes plants grow, too much kills everyone but Noah.

Omega's are all the rage and refer to nothing more than the methyl end of a fatty acid. In Omega 3, the first double bond or cis (unsaturation) lies at the third position from the Methyl (omega end). I'm sure you can gather n-6, and n-9. N-3 includes Alpha-linolenic, an 18 carbon fat, or the prized Eicosapentaenoic (EPA), a 20 carbon fat, and Docosahexaenoic(DHA) a 22 carbon chained fat. N-6 is called Linoleic, Gamma Linolenic, or Arachidonic acid. All except AA are essential.

The ratio we are looking for is 1:1, or 1:2, n-3/n-6. Today some folks are 1:20 or higher. This is simply the effect of the no fat/low fat fad, coupled with partially hydrogenated oils, and processed everything. We try to save money by using cheap food; corn, safflower and soy vegetable oils, and we still pay the price for it.

ALA, or the 18 carbon chain (n-3) fatty acid Alpha-Linoleic acid, is the fat vegetarians tout as their saving grace. It converts to the much more usable and dramatically effective EPA, and DHA. While it's accurate to say ALA does convert but only by a percentage of 40-percent or so. ALA, found in hemp and flax, will not promote health, longevity, anti-inflammatory or any of the benefits EPA, and DHA will. Its really that simple.

Trans fat:
If you want to save a few paragraphs, just don't eat trans fat ... ever.

Now, the trans fats we speak of aren't the natural kind found in incredibly low doses in ruminant (mammal) fats. We're talking about the rightfully demonized man made "plastic fats" found in partially hydrogenated vegetable oils, margarines and shortening.

Trans fats are used in place of "real" fats because they are cheap. They promote shelf life. They provide the same texture as ruminant fat, yet some still fit vegetarian guidelines, they are reusable in restaurant setting, and they seem to taste pretty good.

Trans fats are chemically engineered poly, or monounsaturates that place hydrogen on opposite sides of their molecules, as opposed to the 'cis' reference we made earlier referring to the nature state of hydrogen being on the same side. Since they are adding hydrogen, but not "saturating" it you get "partially hydrogenated".

Added hydrogen reduces the number of double bonds and makes it firmer at room temperature, but permits the sweet melting while baking. If they were completely "hydrogenated" they wouldn't melt, and the less hydrogenation, the more oily the quicker the oxidation.

TF's are like the new kid in school who never seems to fit in. Wherever he hangs out with the other kids he just causes a lot of problems.

Trans fats are a genetic surprise. We have had little more than a couple generations to learn how to behave with them and every study today shows they hurt like a brass knuckle punch to the temple.

Disadvantages to trans fat consumption:

- Lower HDL, and raises LDL, by a dose dependent amount. Meaning we eat a little, a little bad happens, we eat a lot, a lot of bad happens.
- Promotes insulin resistance
- Makes blood stickier
- Weakens cell membrane within the brain
- Lowers testosterone

Dad and I headed to my truck after his doctor's appointment like we'd done every month for 10 years. I hit the metal circle with the cripple on it, he pushed his red walker with the seat several paces behind me. Instead of stutter stepping alongside him like I had an ankle injury, I always hurried our trips by pulling the car around and letting him go it alone.

Today I'd give anything to limp beside him again.

Once in the parking lot he pulled that fiberglass walker to his chest. It weighed ounces, not pounds. When he tried to shoulder and toss it in the truck bed he fell. I watched it from the driver's seat and wondered how a man, not even 60-years-old, was so in need, weak as a child and fragile as a porcelain doll.

Right then and there, while trying to prove a point by letting him do the work he should be able to do, I prayed.

"God, let him get it. Let him understand that he still has a chance and that the responsibility is his not mine, not the doctors. He's fallen and he has to get-up on his own."

The parking brake felt like it was moving in slow motion when I yanked and started to get out to help. I'd hoped for a man embarrassed to have just fallen in front of his son. But like a child unsure of where he was, his blue eyes stared at me from the concrete. I took his hand and steadied him like an unbalanced sack of potatoes.

"Ok," he said with that smile that I'm sure my mom thought was charming three decades ago. "Le ... le ... let's eat."

That was the last time I took my dad to the doctor. He died a month later.

CHAPTER 11

How to Turn Plateaus into Summits

"JB, I need your help," Julie said wearing tears like others wear contacts.

I hear this multiple times a day but not from this girl.

"I have trained with you for four years and never once have I lost motivation," she continued. "Never have I not wanted to workout. I have never ran into a hump that I didn't think I could climb. But lately I just don't want to be here. I don't want to push. I don't want to diet. Whats wrong with me? Have you ever had this happen?"

"Yes, I call it the offseason."

"What do I do to feel better?," she asked. "I know if I stop I will eventually come back, but it will be so much harder. I still love it and all, but I just don't like it right now."

"Julie, there's no perfect answer. The more we search for perfection the harder it is to feel good. That's why you're experiencing your offseason right now, you're so attached to perfection you won't allow yourself good. You're so focused on where you're going you can't be proud of where you've been."

She cried.

Some think it's silly to shed a tear over a workout and food, but when you make health a lifestyle it's scary to think of life without it. Especially when your passion becomes your burden.

I went on dissecting Julie's life with her, trying to draw correlations between her story and the many that have come before her. She was getting married soon, the summer was over and she recently returned to teaching and coaching high school basketball. Her honeymoon was over and she wasn't too far past a competition she had done very well in.

Julie had begun to let the things in her life run her, not the other way around. A constant need for perfection and approval of those she respects wasn't helping the situation either.

The Offseason

Seasons change no matter the consistency at which you lead your life. Seasons of growth, spiritual or otherwise. Seasons of despair, of joy. These are inevitable and productive if we are willing to look at what those seasons are teaching us as opposed to letting them throw us off the path. All seasons can be productive except for one; "The Offseason."

For 12-16 weeks I worked out two and three times a day. I would eat far less calories than I burned. I watched the mirror like children watch their favorite cartoon. I was getting ready for a stage. A stage where everyone would judge me and the work I was putting in. I was tired, but motivated. I had a plan and while every single day was far from glorious, the goal kept me focused.

Admirable as this dedication is, the reason for it isn't. The reason I had to work so hard was because I believed health was a part time job, not a lifetime profession. You treat your home a lot different when you finally become an owner, not a tenant.

I was a bodybuilder. I trained every day yet a simple trip up the stairs would leave me out of breath. I entered my first offseason when I graduated high school at 5'8" 120 pounds. By the time I was 22 years old, I weighed 260 pounds.

My Offseason was a hiding place.

Prevention

We don't have to be fortune tellers to see what's coming. Simply take a long look at your past combined with a hard look at your present. Why were you successful? Why aren't you anymore? What do you really want? How are you different?

There is no Super Bowl in life, no championship, no medals. Even if we're getting beat, or old, or bored, we must never leave the race.

1. Write down what you want out of the week. What good things you expect.
2. Extrapolate that to a month making sure to place all the other things in the timeline that you know may add to your plate, just so they won't surprise you. We have enough surprises as it is.
3. Make a monthly goal that can be added together to make a three month goal. Personally, anything more is very difficult for my " ADD" rattled mind. I may have future goals and dreams that don't change for sometime, but the methods that get me there certainly do.
4. Do inventory. It's not all about future steps, it's also about past achievements. I often look at pictures of the happiest times I have had competing with my friends. I look back at my journals and read how I felt and revel in the person I am, the person who I came from

being. I regularly sit and just chat with someone I am helping to ensure I am focusing on them because if I focus on myself I will always let myself down.

This inventory helps me to stay the path making sure that even if I do hit a plateau void of motivation, my memories can help me through, not just my goals.

5. Victory loves preparation and I prepare to be let down by others, and myself. My whole life people have lied to me and let me down, I expect nothing different out of a broken race I am very much a part of. This isn't negative, this is positively the only way I can function everyday without letting the roadblocks of people cut me off. Without letting my own goals become my vices. Without letting my internal need for perfection overtake my need for progression. It's not about you or others walking perfectly, it's about walking. Sometimes all we can do is limp along the outskirts.

6. A never ending timeline that you have in your sight regularly staring you in the face takes minutes to create and will prevent many of these feeling from coming up. If it takes too long to produce goals and prospects we won't do them ... at least I know I won't.

    For instance, this month I wrote "I want to PR my hundred meter swim by 10 full seconds," on my timeline. It sat right beside adding more variety to my food. After I write these down, maybe I pick another one about a specific book and a page I want to be by the end of next week.

These constant, small, meaningful goals make it so easy to stay constantly in-season. I tend to round them out like this but you do as you like;

1. Spiritual. "Reading three chapters of the bible every time I open it. Opening it everyday"
2. Writing. "Forcing myself to write about things for an hour a day that will benefit others for the first time that I have wrote and described for the millionth time."

3. Diet. "Trying a different cooking method over the weekends that I may be able to pass on to another. Trying to gain a pound of muscle this week. Trying to lose two pounds of fat next week."
4. Workout. "Twice a week for 10 minutes at a time-playing on the rings. Walking on my hands for 300' over the course of the week"
5. Others. "Sending an email everyday just to tell someone good job."

The key to these goals is that I set new ones before I achieve old ones.

The key item to living in-season is to constantly put things on the list that need checking off. Once there is nothing to check off, you're officially in the offseason

Treatment
But alas, you're already there, huh?

You're in that offseason you say. You either did all the above and it just didn't work, or you didn't and now you're screwed, left dreading what you once loved. Fine, next time plan better.

While you may not like the way to climb out of the pit, the goal is still to get out. So like it or not, pissed off or not, just start doing something or you'll end up content doing nothing.

1. Change it all, no matter how trivial
Your laser-like focus has become a swamp of disinterest. You feel lost in the ocean below the narrow bridge you fell from. You feel "spread thin," not "dialed in." You need something different.

You need everything to be different

Focus on the things that are guaranteed to add vibrance to your life. Diet, workouts, friends and such. Focus on them, but unlike you ever have before.

You will find that you can't travel the same burnt bridge twice. Once you have used one avenue for joy and progress, and unfortunately regressed, it becomes necessary to take a new path. After all, you are a new human.

- Drive a different way to work than yesterday
- Workout at a different time
- Workout with different people
- Perform only the workouts you like. It's no time to be beat down by your weaknesses, it's time to be built up by your strengths
- Run more than lift
- Lift more than run
- Eat something unusual, yet still something good for you
- Find someone new to eat with, so you can educate them as well as solidify yourself
- Meditate
- Workout less and ensure they are absolutely productive workouts
- Don't miss these crucial workout times
- Focus on the mirror
- Focus on the bar.

Turn everything on its head. Flip the coin until it comes back up winner enough times to put this offseason behind you.

Always remember; "Familiarity breed contempt."

*Seriously, pick one of these and do it.

2. Everything is victory

If we celebrate every victory today, even if it really isn't comparable to a victory yesterday, we will get back in season faster. Recognize and applaud every forward step you take today no matter how small. Eventually, they will lead you where you want to go. Eventually, that quicksand will release its hold if we remain thankful for every breath.

3. The Cobweb

After basking in the smallest victory, look around and become aware of why you forget those "W"" so fast. The cobwebs of our daily activities frequently rob us of our joy before we are aware. If your life's cobweb has found a huge season of growth, adjust your gaze and open your eyes. Remember, a yacht looks big in a lake, but small in the ocean.

If your cobweb of life is bigger than it was a few months ago, and a looming achievement has come and gone unrealized, take heart in the fact that you have a cobweb at all. Remember, tedious times will give way to flourishing events as soon as we are content with trying and failing … repeatedly.

We call our mistakes experience. Times in our lives where we didn't plan enough to be better is called an "offseason". We call ourselves weak for feeling lonely or indifferent. Weariness sets in when we cannot let go of our arbitrary notions of perfection and the limitations it creates.

While constantly trying to be perfect we miss out on good.

Julie walked away after much discussion and found a way. As uncomfortable as it may have been, she had a plan.

The point isn't always moving in the perfect direction, the point is moving.

Once, Julie remembered that, she again found the comfort she had been missing. With a new twist on her tried and true passions, Julie viewed what was once old as if it were new again. Constant progress creates new waves that leave us motivated for eternity, while treading water leads us nowhere, tired and ready to go back to the shore.

CHAPTER 12

BUTTER AND COCONUT

Not long ago my phone rang to the tune of all damn day.

A pissed parent of a young athlete had a bone to pick, a bone that sounded a lot like "sue you for everything you've got."

The story goes as stories do. Well meaning coach meets wide eyed youth and discerning parental figure who isn't really listening, thinking, "what's this gonna cost me."

Well meaning coach, explains passion for helping folks, discerning parent, having been raised up as many of us have, lied to and manipulated by the media, hears passions but thinks "sales pitch." Who can blame them?

Begrudgingly, discerning parent gives into the cravings of a youth who wants to throw the ball farther. Who knows, maybe we can get a free ride?

It's like Mario vs Donkey Kong; Parents beat their chests and coaches coach.

Maybe the parent was a heyday athlete and they think they know better. Maybe they're out of shape and your very appearance makes them feel self conscious. Maybe they think you will hurt their child. Whatever the case the reactions are the same. The parent masks their hostility with a barrage of questions and waits for an answer they dislike so they can feel better when they fire you.

This rage stems from their hatred, or at least annoyance, with their current lot in life. Not only do they see the passion I deliver which they write off as manipulation, but they see the muscles, clear skin, small waist and smile … all something they have long traded in for Sunday's on the couch, evenings with a beer, and pasta for dinner.

"Are you trying to kill my boy," the concerned mom said when I finally called her back.

"Is he injured?"

"You told him to eat butter and coconut. I read on the internet that those are saturated fats. Then I called my doctor and asked his opinion. He said the reason we have margarine is so we can stay away from all that. Are you trying to give my son a heart attack? I should sue you."

Whew, I thought it was something worth a damn. I thought he blew an ACL, tore a rotator, got a girlfriend pregnant because he has abs.

"I understand your concern, Pam (name changed), but I assure you he will not die of a heart attack. In fact I'm sure if he did eat what I recommended and you had his biomarkers checked, as I recommended when we started, he would be just fine".

"Yeah, my doctor said the only people who can eat like that and not die are those people with really good genetics, and you must have that because you still have muscles and stuff. If you were like me you would be fat or worse," she said trailing off like a 10-year-old arguing with a bigger badder adult.

"I bet your doctor's fat," I said before thinking.

"My doctor is so busy helping everyone he doesn't have the time to workout like you and those people you hang out with. And he has genetics like me."

I swelled like a balloon about to pop, my chest peacocked and I drew in one of those underwater breaths, the kind you take when you're on dry ground and ready to give someone several earfuls without stopping.

"Maybe the parent was a heyday athlete and they think they know better. Maybe they're out of shape and your very appearance makes them feel self conscious. Maybe they think you will hurt their child. Whatever the case the reactions are the same. The parent masks their hostility with a barrage of questions and waits for an answer they dislike so they can feel better when they fire you."

Then something happened. Before I breathed fire, I thought that maybe we really we're both on the same side. One of us just had the right info. I started to think of Pam as a less than confident average American who wants the best for her kids.

My job isn't to judge Pam, or be mad at her, it's education without anger.

"Pam, do you read all I write on my blog, all the time I put in, all the research?" I asked.

"Who has time for that nonsense?" she replied.

"Well, Pam, I urge you to read some links that I would be more than happy to send you."

"If you send me anything, or talk to my son again, I will sue you," Pam said before she hung up the phone.

Thankfully these exchanges are not the norm. Frequently, in fact, folks believe me and others like me, they just can't make the jump from belief to action.

I want Pam's picture in the back of your mind when I ask you to engage in two specific activities within this chapter.

"My job isn't to judge Pam, or be mad at her, it's education without anger."

I'm going to ask you to try something new, often. Something different, and hopefully be blessed for it. I want you to try something completely sideways of what the media is selling and I want you to become something completely different than what the media creates. Media creates hype, turmoil, speculation. I just want you to feel better.

Eat Coconut

Coconut is Saturated Fat. See below for the benefits of SF from our fat chapter.

SF Benefits:

- Your heart muscle works better. Yup the heart prefers saturated fat more than any organ around.
- Saturated fat raises HDL(high density lipids).
- Cell walls become stronger.
- Improve gut health, stimulate gut fighting bacteria. Specifically the MCT's in coconut. These little wonders ward off offending agents in our stomachs due to the lauric acid.
- Drastically improve bone health. While calcium plays a role in bone health, it's much more about eating the foods that promote its absorption, and not eating the foods that don't. Specifically, we would do well to ensue 50-percent of our total fat intake be saturated. That way, we can create an environment for proper calcium absorption, and therefore healthy bones.

- Improves Omega 3 absorption. Yup Omega 3 is a polyunsaturated fat, but without its brother the saturated fat, it cannot bring the party to the party goers. Not to mention the fact that the more Saturated fat you eat, the less you need Omega 3.
- Makes you lean. The more fat you eat, the less of everything else. The more fat you eat, the better you become at burning it.

A little on Coconut:

Coconut oil -- butter, flakes, water, cream, and milk -- are about as saturated as it gets. But it's not just about the amount of hydrogen contained, it's about the particular properties of coconut that make it so appealing. In fact, I ingest some form of coconut in every meal and I have prescribed it for the past decade. Even before I knew all the reason why.

Back in my bodybuilding days we were told to take coconut because it helped you lean out, we did, it did. When you're 20-years-old results are king, reasons are time consuming.

Today coconut has found its way back into the kitchens of Americans everywhere. This is a stark difference from a couple decades ago when Coconut was demonized as a "tropical fat" and paired with Keys and his seven countries study. To Keys, coconut is one of the main culprits behind heart disease.

The lipid hypothesis turned a nation against fat, especially tropical fats that were used heavily in the 60's and 70's. This also happens to be the time when trans fats were becoming in-vogue, and much cheaper. Convenient how media timed events coordinate with enterprise timed profits ... nothing is coincidence.

MCT

Coconut fat contains the highest percentage of medium chain triglycerides when compared to other fat sources. Most fats we ingest, like Omega's and Monounsaturates, are long chained fatty acids. Meaning they have a carbon chain that begins around 18 carbon atoms, and continues up to 22 carbon atoms.

Medium chain fatty acids sit right around 12 carbons in length. The length of the carbon chain generally describes the rate at which it will leave the system, or become fully digested. For instance, EPA is 18 carbons atoms in length and stays in the system much longer than MCT, making fat variety essential to optimal survival.

The simplest way to explain MCT is fat that cannot be converted to fat. Not easily anyway. In fact the amount you would have to eat would be more than your stomach could handle, speaking of course as someone who has tried ingesting too much MCT oil.

MCT oil acts as a carbohydrate when speaking in terms of a preferential energy source. Coconut is an energy substrate meaning they are first in line to be burned as fuel. If your low carb living like we recommend this is exactly what you want. Not only will MCT satisfy Leptin so you won't be hungry, but they will be the first to burn leaving protein for muscle building.

Like alcohol, MCT from coconut bypasses the stomach digestion requiring no bile for absorption, or breakdown. Therefore, Medium chain triglycerides are a great choice of fat for folks without a gallbladder, celiacs, or crohn's. MCT oil will bypass the lymphatic system unlike other fats and become absorbed directly into our bloodstream where it is used as energy.

MCT gives us the immediate energy of a carbohydrate without the insulin spike of glucose. MCT adds calories to performance without the chance of a calorie spillover leading to weight gain, which admittedly is hard anyway if there are not carbohydrates present. The question isn't "should, I", or "shouldn't, I". The question is "how much?"

Additional Coconut benefits:
Coconut is saturated fat and specifically helps us absorb essentially fats like Omega-3.

Coconut oil is stable at room temperature and since it's saturated with hydrogen it doesn't go rancid. In fact its smoke point is great for cooking unlike olive oil.

Coconut raises HDL and Lowers LDL, unlike many made plastic fats, or PUFA's like Omega-6.

Coconut can be consumed by folks that have had a cholecystectomy (gallbladder removed). MCT oil is absorbed through the small intestine and does not need bile from the gallbladder to emulsify

Coconut improves insulin sensitivity.

Coconut contains lauric acid. When converted to monolaurin it is the antiviral, antibacterial, and antiprotozoal improving gut health drastically.

Coconut fights lipid coated viruses like HIV, Herpes, Influenza

Coconut makes you leaner.

Coconut Culprits:
Coconut water serves many purposes from a great addition to a lean individuals post workout shake, to electrolyte replacement. But as a general rule it still contains too much sugar. Most of us should avoid this.

Coconut Milk, whole not lite, in and of itself may be ok, but the amount generally called for in recipes is more than we require as health humans. Best avoided.

Sweetened coconut is also taking hold because of the wealth of literature promoting coconut today. And once any food is good for you, it also gets sugar added so addiction keeps us in the checkout line.

Stick with the basics:

Unsweetened coconut flakes
Coconut Oil
MCT oil
Coconut butter

#2 Eat Ghee

Ghee is a super concentrated form of butterfat. If you were to cook out all milk proteins and sugars you would end up with a super stable long lasting fat source with a smoke point nearing 500 degrees.

Butter contains casein proteins which is a gut irritant to humans. Ghee solves the butter problem by skimming out the solids and contaminants leaving only the butterfat.

Ghee Benefits:

- Quality source of Vitamins A, D, E, and K. The fat soluble ones.
- The specific fatty profile aids in the absorption of other nutrients.
- The butyric acid is anti-viral adding to proper gut health, again providing an unhampered environment for mental and physical wellness.
- Fat makes you full.
- Smoke point of at least 450 degrees.
- Everything else positive listed in our fat chapters and above.

After I wrote this I was motivated to check in with Pam and her kid ... from the legal protection of a computer screen and Facebook account of course.

I searched her Facebook profile and found her throwing another personal trainer fit. Apparently she had enlisted the help of a coach for herself. And apparently he'd told her some of the same things I'd told her son.

The ones like Pam are the most confusing. What would I have to gain by telling you to eat coconut? I don't own Hawaii. For that matter, what would I have to gain by giving the wrong information?

It's not even faith I'm asking from Pam and people like her, it's common sense. We get fat because of bad choice not genetics. We stay that way because changing is admitting we were wrong.

CHAPTER 13

How to Fast

"Listen dude, I did your whole Breakfast is Bad thing, but not eating for 24 hours!? I'm not muslim, jewish, catholic or any other religion that says I shouldn't eat for a full day. I'm American and I get hungry a couple hours after every meal, let alone a whole day."

Derrick was 25-pounds smaller than we we met and said he felt great.

"Have I let you down, yet?," I asked.

"No, but I remember a few years ago you told people to eat seven meals a day and that breakfast was the most important part. Next year you'll say fasting is worthless while you experiment on me."

"Touche," I said.

Derrick was a triathlete at the time, wanting to "break the seal" he called it, and before he turned forty. Sort of an athlete's mid-life crisis. He looked at me like you look at your mom when she said "because I said so."

"Fine, but when I get hungry, I'm calling you," he said.

You're Not Jesus:
Remember when Jesus fasted in the desert while tempted by Satan?

Thankfully you're not the Messiah and the sort of fasting we'll describe and advocate will last no longer than 24-hours at any given time.

Jesus, Buddha, Gandhi; all fasted for much longer than we will. As they, and others like them have proven, the body can function for weeks without food.

Fasting takes advantage of hormones and it isn't religiously owned or fad inspired. Fasting is ancient. Fasting is old fashioned.

One of our biggest plagues besetting mankind today is ingenuity. Our inability to be inconvenienced. There is a fast food drive-way on every corner, a convenience store on every street. Fasting was our ancestors way of fighting illness, staying lean, having energy and getting things done.

However ancestral famine wasn't programmed, it was forced. The benefits weren't studied they were realized. The feast was fleeting while the famine was lasting and they most assuredly reaped the rewards. Most likely, unhappily.

Long term fasts may be productive and healing but so are short term ones. And when done correctly, they have zero discomfort and may even add to our enjoyment of daily life.

"Fasting takes advantage hormones and it isn't religiously owned or fad inspired. Fasting is ancient. Fasting is old fashioned."

I read a study that summed it up perfectly. A group of mice fasted for five days. All their health markers improved. But the doctors noted one "odd" thing. The mice seemed depressed.

The scientists made a change.

The mice went 24, 48 and 72-hours without food. Most of the same benefits from the longer fast above were realized, and the mice seemed fine (I have no clue how they measure micey moods). Interestingly, from 24 to 72-hours, the benefits stalled. It seemed the sweet spot for fasting, was 18 - 24-hours.

The Media Has More To Do With Your Metabolism:
Unfortunately we're all twisted up by commercials, billboards, and pop-ups that do nothing more than seduce us into believing we need to eat every few hours. In fact, today, it's a widespread, albeit incorrect, theory that eating small frequent meals burns more fat than eating less frequent bigger meals. What a scam for the companies making the 4000 calories per American per day.

Did you ever wonder why Subway, Starbucks and Taco Bell serve breakfast now? Why Taco Bell and Wendy's stay open late and have fourth, fifth, and sixth meals?

Metabolism is a funny thing when it comes to media and our representation. Our metabolism is not some hallowed object we were either blessed or cursed with at birth. "He can eat that because his metabolism is so fast." Or, "wait until her metabolism slows down, then her butt won't look that anymore."

These statements cloud good judgement and regale all hard work to a crapshoot based on good or bad genetics. Your metabolism is nothing but chemical reactions happening in your body right now. And the simplest way to change the expression is to change the drugs.

If you're currently eating the Standard American Diet then you will need to eat every 2-3 hours to feel comfortable. Living on glucose is like cheap gas that burns off too fast leaving you in need of a fill up.

Converting the system to a fat metabolism and your energy levels out, hunger subsides and you get lean.

Calories in or calories out

Around 480 BC Spartans fought back the Persians. They feared oppression and unjust governing and loss of freedom. Today our Persians are the food industry and they're much more stealthy and aggressive.

If the Spartans are yelling, "It's the kind of calorie that matters," the Persians would be screaming "No, it's the amount." And frequently, as in times of war, both sides are right, and both are wrong.

Xerxes only wanted to unite a world under his order, have them govern and worship on their own, and get the taxes for defending them. Spartans wanted freedom and were powerful enough to demand it.

The Persians would argue that we can eat whatever we want as long as we follow the rules of thermodynamics, meaning as long as we burn more than we eat we will lose weight. In theory this sounds great, but we are not machines and we don't respond as such.

Years ago, as a competitive bodybuilder, I was ordered by my trainer at the time to disprove the Calorie in vs Calories out conundrum. I gave up 300 calories worth of oats in exchange for 300 calories of fruit. That was the only change. In three weeks time I weighed 5.3-pounds more. Nothing else changed, I ate the same thing everyday and trained as close to the same as possible.

Weight watchers, Jenny Craig and all the other calorie counter programs are selling a fat gaining lie. Do you immediately lose weight? Yes - muscle.

"Metabolism is a funny thing when it comes to media and our representation. Our metabolism is not some hallowed object we were either blessed or cursed with at birth. "He can eat that because his metabolism is so fast". Or, "wait until her metabolism slows down, then her butt won't look that anymore."

Having more muscle burns more fat. This is why worrying only about the amount of calories fails. This is why we focus on the kind of calories as well as the amount.

After a long day of killing his enemies, a Spartan would return home for what would prove to be his one basic meal of the day. It would consist of meat, fat and maybe veggies (black soup was actually their main dish consisting of pig parts blood and salt). He would eat until his portion was gone.

Our warrior ancestors would not have had a little piece of cake that was only 200 calories, he would have ingested 1000 calories of wild boar. One sends insulin through the roof and primes our system to gain fat, the other primes the system to burn fat. One is a hunter, the other is prey.

I'm sure you've heard, "too much of a good thing." This counts with food also. Just because 30 oz of protein a day is awesome, doesn't mean 50 oz is better. It's all about manipulating our hormones so they function best.

For instance, overeating protein ends in excessive glucose production from the liable glycogenic amino acids. Overeating fat gives us more energy than we need. Too much energy is stored as fat for later. When there is enough energy consumed we stay the same. When there is too little energy consumed from the right sources we lose fat.

How To Fast:

1. First, begin by entering Ketosis as described within this book. After you have removed the carbohydrates and created the environment that wants to burn stored body fat because there is no sugar around, fasting will feel easier that eating.

2. Drink water. Half your bodyweight in ounces per day is a great basal water intake. Ketosis produces ketone bodies and fatty waste that desperately needs to be excreted. Becoming dehydrated is no way to be healthy, let alone thin or active.

3. As we mentioned in our breakfast is for losers chapter, eating right after getting outta bed is silly; don't.

   Your first fast will be from your last meal in the evening to your first meal of the following day, which should be well over 5 hours of wake time. For instance:

   Last meal=8pm
   Rise=6am
   first meal=11am
   Fasted time not including digestion=15 hours

Now that more like a 10 hour fast because we are in a fed state for about 5 hours after eating, but it still counts in close to the same manner as fasting the full 15 hours. The best thing is the bulk of the fast was while we were sleeping.

4. Simply start adding three hours to your first fast every week thereafter until you reach a 24 hour period without food. Then, if you feel up to it, don't start the clock on fasting until four hours after your last meal. This ensures almost the entire 24 hours was in a fasted state, not just food-less.

   After your 12-15-24 hour fast has ended, eat a normal meal, no gorging.

   But you shouldn't need to anyway. Remember during this fast your body fed you with body fat.

   The first meal should be enjoyable and really no different than any other. In fact, many folks look forward to their weekly or bi-weekly fast because of the freedom and energy created by not worrying about food, and by properly activating our ancestral hormones.

"Your metabolism is nothing but chemical reactions happening in your body right now. And the simplest way to change the expression is to change the drugs."

5. Journal your feelings and your day. Even the best intentions are hampered without proper data. If your first fast was after a horrible night's sleep it's safe to say this will be a disaster. It's good to know you slept poorly so you can make an honest assessment of your efforts, not a brazen blame game because you missed your juice.

Should I workout fasted

I heard you fire-breathing athletes losing your mind when this chapter began. In fact, I was against fasting for more years than I would like to admit because of a misplaced fear of diminished performance returns.

Fasting was just one of the many systems I wrote off as mythology while disregarding biology. I used to think I would lose muscle and gain fat if I did not eat seven times a day. Let alone forgoing food for half a day or more.

Some of us feel a bit anxious or nauseous the first time we workout fasted. There are a few supplements that are either making this worse, or supplements that can make it better, but it could be nothing more than a heightened sense of awareness you have yet to ever truly experience. It could be your caveman side shining through.

It would be foolish to believe you would immediately feel amazing switching your entire body chemistry back to the way it works best. If you have been living one way your entire life, regardless of if it's optimal or not, the body still establishes a set point like a thermostat.

The anxiety or butterflies you feel in your stomach when you workout fasted is your nervous system. Be it the Autonomic, or Enteric. It's nerves that makes us function, and when they aren't digesting food, they are wired to go nuts. Nuts during a workout is what you want. But if nuts isn't your normal, it will feel like you're gonna throw up.

Back in our breakfast chapter we spoke about the circadian rhythm. When we get out of bed after sleeping preferably 10-hours or so, we are functioning within the sympathetic nervous system. Potentially cortisol is higher than it will be in the evening. This is a good thing. This means we are wired to defend. Eating turns that off. Eating shifts us into a parasympathetic nervous system to help digest the food currently consumed. This is why large meals make us sleepy.

Assuming you have eliminated the majority of carbohydrates, it still may take some time to feel comfortable working out fasted, but it's worth it.

Even if your workouts are in the evening you can still work out fasted without having to fast the entire day. Simply eat a meal more than 6 hours before your workout, pretty much guaranteeing you will be in a fasted state when you workout even if it's evening.

Two-a-dayers
The only adjustment I would make is for athletes engaging in more than one workout in a day.

Those folks eating the Paleo diet we recommend will have a glycogen and energy refill optimal for another workout in about 24-hours. Those athletes wanting dirty, nasty performance multiple times in a 24-hour period will need carbohydrates to top the tank off quicker. If you're that guy, employ something akin to the recovery shake below:

Multiple Workout Day Recovery meal:
14 oz Coconut Water
20 gram whey protein
Sweet potato

Suspicious Supplements

Caffeine is a staple in my daily life but caffeine is a stimulant. Before we started fasting, most of us had some type of food on our stomachs when we had our morning cup of Joe. When fasting, coffee usually enters the system all by itself, and you're already in the "fight" version of fight or flight, and adding more fire to the fight may be too much for you to control.

If you're still killing seven cups of Starbucks a day and fasting feels like a roller coaster, cut way back and feel way better.

Green Tea is another very popular, lightish stimulant. Most of us should be fine with some but it still bears mention If you're taking this supplement and feel edgy, stop it while fasting.

Ibuprofen and other NSAIDs are something I am ok with when the time is right ... but the time is rarely right.

Stupendous Supplements:

Glutamine is a glycogenic amino acid we have spoken about before. Think, bridge over the carb free choppy water until you get to the carb-less shore. Without the bridge the journey may still be possible, with the bridge rough waters seem tame.

Introduce glutamine while fasting at no more than 15 grams per day, broken into three separate doses. Reduce by 5 grams or so until you no longer need it.

L-Carnitine, among other things, helps initiate the mitochondrial shift. Basically, it makes the transition from sugar metabolism to fat metabolism go down a little faster and more comfortable.

To make this process smoother, and to give you more energy, take 500mg of LC a day, reducing by 100 mg each week until your out.

Gymne Sylvester is a leaf that folks have chewed for some time to prevent sweet cravings. It is sold in pill form but works in pure form as well. The leaves kind of ruin your taste buds for a bit making sweet food taste bitter and unappealing. The active compound in this supplement suppresses the craving from within and can be a good addition for those sweet lovers out there.

Magnesium is yet another must for many of us today. From sleep management to a true source of healthy bones, magnesium is much more a regulator of longevity than we give it credit for. Take magnesium before bed, preferably with Zinc, 400-600mg per day.

Zinc is involved in just about every process within the body. Take 30 mg per day.

Vitamin "D"- Sun in a bottle. Testosterone mapper, fat burner, Anti-inflammatory, insulin sensitivity and much more. In fact "D" is not even a Vitamin, but a hormone. 2000-5000 iu per day.

Omega 3 (n-3, Fish Oil, EPA, DHA, PUFA's) - Never go a day without it. Our diets are full of far too much Omega-6 which is not inherently bad, but the drastic ratio change from our prehistoric friends is one of the main reasons our health waivers today. Ensure a n-3/n-6 ratio of 1/2, or 1/4, not the average american of 1/30. Shoot for .5, up to 1.5 grams per 10 lbs of bodyweight per day.

Water processes metabolic waste and rids the body of excessive ketones. It's not really a supplement but supplements don't work if you're dehydrated

Nuun is a wonderful source of electricity. Have you ever heard of marathon runners crossing the finish line chugging water right into a heart attack? This doesn't mean they were dehydrated, this means they were imbalanced. Electrolyte imbalance to be exact.

Many runners drink enough H2o but miss the salt. They become hyponatremic. This is how too much water kills people. After all, the body, especially the heart, is run by electrical impulses in its most basic form. Destroy any part of the basis for your internal electrical conduction and depression, cramping, and muscle sprains are just the beginning.

Caffeine is an odd recommendation, right? Especially when it's on the suspicious list. Remember, the reason to avoid caffeine was because it made you as paranoid as a terrorist at an airport. If, however, you find yourself a little mentally foggy and energy deprived, drink black coffee and see if that natural jolt doesn't eliminate brain fog.

The phone call
Derrick called me after his first day fasting. Actually, he called my while fasting and like any caring coach, I ignored him and called him that evening.

"So how was it?," I asked.

"I called you earlier, the hell can't you answer your phone?," he said.

"Busy; how was it?"

"I almost chewed my arm off."

After Derrick complained for another minute or so I cut him off.

"You weren't starving, you were bored," I said. "I bet you annoyed everyone around you because your were so go-go. I bet everyone irritated you, and not because you were hungry, because they couldn't keep up."

The phone got quiet, Derrick clicked a pen or something waiting for me to continue. I kept typing on my computer.

"I hate you," he said.

"You're welcome."

One month later, and a few more fun phone calls, and Derrick "broke the seal." He was the leanest and fastest he'd ever been.

Fasting isn't for everyone.

Some people can actually die from intense exercise. Some will die if they eat fruit. Others get sick when they don't eat. The point is; never be afraid to go against the grain. My friend, and many others including myself, have to learn the hard way. But at least there are those of us still willing to learn. The last 10 years of my life have proven this adage more true than I could ever imagine;

The more I know, the more I realize, I know nothing.

The more I experiment, the more freedom I find in the oddest places.

CHAPTER 14

NORMAL VS COMMON

"**I**'m just looking to tone."

This is how I met Janet. All 5' 6" of just-like-everyone-else.

"I mean the abs that these others girls have don't really interest me."

Wrinkles were creeping along each side of Janet's face like tiny insect legs crawling from her hair. Short, dark hair that looked like it had been cut with a hatchet,

"Just last week my doctor said I'm totally fine, but I still wouldn't mind to lose a pound or two, and firm the fat around the back of my arm … and butt … oh, and that area where your butt and leg meet - the 'bu-thigh.' I hate that."

Janet was the Alpha of her bridge club. The grandma who could pass for the mom. The one the conservative ladies loved talking about.

I liked Janet right away.

It's cool to watch people take the hardest step right in front of you. The first one.

She had done her research, she knew the results she wanted and they could be achieved at my gym. The one with all the scantily clad females in tight shorts and males with tattoos and no shirts. Thankfully, this is only part of our diverse population, but admittedly, one that is intimidating.

The logical person says, "clearly what they're doing is working, I will go there." The emotional person, who we all are at the worst time says, "I need to be in shape before I go or they will laugh at me. Or I might die."

Let me ask you this: Do you think a fat person, who doesn't want to be fat anymore, would be better off hanging with fat people or fit people?

It's weird but when the only cure is discomfort we look to be comfortable, caged again with all the other species just like us. When we rationalize intuition it's no longer intuition … its justification.

"So your ab-offended," I said.

"Well no, I just don't wanna look like her," she replied pointing to one of our fit girls slamming her chest on the ground as if a bomb was about to go off, immediately rebounding like a basketball with gleaming abs pulled from the cover of Muscle Fitness - minus the air brushing. It's called a burpee

Janet's statement didn't shock me, I'd heard it before, I just didn't believe it.

I mean who hates abs, firm muscles and a tight butt? And all at 47-years-old with impeccable biomarkers and an injury free machine? Exactly! No-one.

The goal of this book is to present the truth through nutrition. But nutrition doesn't begin with your digestive system, nutrition begins with your mind. If your mind is jacked, so is your nutrition, and if 97% of all diseases and cancers are preventable through proper drug intake (food), then we better start with our heads.

"Let me ask you this: Do you think a fat person, who doesn't want to be fat anymore, would be better off hanging with fat people or fit people?"

Working out and eating well is simply a function of a healthy mind.

"Janet, did you look around the waiting room the last time you were at your doctor's office?," I asked.

"Yes. I have to wait every time I arrive because there are so many people waiting before me."

"What was your honest opinion of those waiting with you?"

She stumbled and began to speak softly, "they were fat."

The Doctor Dogma

Doctors, like the one Janet goes too, build practices around what we are willing and unwilling to do. If we were willing to exercise a lot and eat for performance, they would prescribe it. But we're not.

The next option is a pill that lengthens our lives and treats symptoms. If that's all we're willing to do, why would they prescribe anything else?

As a whole, doctors gain nothing from nutritional knowledge. If they did, barely legible prescriptions pads would read: Eat meat, nuts, seeds, green vegetables and coconut.

Common isn't healthy, just look around

The herd mentality is in our DNA.

Our nature may very well be to follow the leader and join the masses in a hodgepodge of poorly defined statistics. Just because our biomarkers look like our neighbors and their neighbors, and so on, doesn't mean we should be comfortable. In fact, like Janet, we should be asking: What's healthy? What's optimal?

When I asked Janet about the patients she hangs out with in that sterile waiting room full of two-year-old Sports Illustrated and out of date Home and Garden magazines, she began to question her diagnose. The scary one thats says, "Congratulations you're just like everyone else."

The "common" Fasting Blood Glucose for a 30-year-old is 80% more likely to make you diabetic in 10 years. The common diet of high carbs and low fat has produced a national epidemic of obesity. Common is the enemy of optimal and the bridge to optimal is uncomfortable. Uncomfortable, but well worth the trip.

Health Markers and Twinkie's:
Common vs Optimal is explained beautifully in a diet once adopted and publicized heavily by accredited nutritionist Mark Haub.

Haub's principle experiment was eating only Little Debbies, Twinkies, and the like. Haubs contention was that as long as he burned more calories than what he consumed he would lose wieght. He did.

Haubs reduced his body-fat by nearly 10%, taking him down to 24% overall. Haubs also experienced a so called improvement in his cholesterol numbers. His HDL (good cholesterol) jumped up 20-percent, while his LDL (bad cholesterol) dropped 20-percent.

But before you rush out to the Kwik-E-Mart like I wanted to do, read what Haubs has to say about his results.

"Does that mean I'm healthier? Or does it mean something about how we define health. That we're missing something?" - Haubs

Yes, eating less calories plays a significant role in health, but what we eat matters more.

Interestingly, the experiment only measured two strings from a huge quilt. Remember in our cholesterol chapter, we need all parts of the equation to get the right answer.

"Common is the enemy of optimal and the bridge to optimal is uncomfortable."

It would have been nice to see Mark's H1Ac, FBG, Triglycerides, C-reactive Protein, and Vit-D before and after. Not just the two biomarkers that are almost guaranteed to go down in the face of less meat eating, and more carbohydrate ingestion.

Thermodynamically, if we burn the equivalent of 2,400 Calories per day, we will lose weight if we were to only ingest 1,800 calories, right? But if you recall from various chapters, things aren't always so black and white.

For instance, even while in a Calorie deficient state, 300 Calories of candy acts a lot differently than 300 Calories of coconut. Humans are a ball of hormones and hormones don't seem to fit into our little equations all the time.

Starving, Surviving or Thriving:
I have faith in the fact that most us will make our way back to optimal living. On our way the media will continue its roadblocks, news will come up with the next thing to fear, and pharmacies will invent the next pill we just have to take.

Hopefully we learn to read "studies show" as "he who had the most money and got the results he paid for."

I feel sorry for doctors like the ones above. How can they help a world unwilling to help itself? How can they cure common?

Our greatest fear in life should be growing up to be just like everybody else.

CHAPTER 15

EVERYDAY DRUGS

When I adventure through my library I ride with Alexander.

I fight with Leonidas.

I shake the hand of Tyler Durden and then punch him in the face.

I sit and listen to Jesus.

Even if you're not religious, the sermon on the mount is a precious way to live. A beautiful way to be, forgotten by everyone of us at one point or another.

⅄

No sooner had he finished his address than a cigarette was burning and coffee poured in his honor. He left the stage and returned to the tent reserved for guest speakers.

This particular event found me as the resident food expert. I often find myself in the midst of doctors, professors and guru's. It's especially endearing when everybody has letters behind their name except me. My introduction is; "Please welcome, Josh Bunch ... (uncomfortable silence) he's gonna talk about food."

At this particular venue I was part of the talent volunteering time to help raise money for charity. The other guy didn't answer his phone.

I had already said my piece and figured, since I didn't get shot for saying milk is bad, and I wasn't assassinated by Monsanto for bad-mouthing grains, it was a good day. Until one man spoke.

This particular speaker/smoker was an expert on how to give up addiction. He was a ten year recovering alcoholic who owned his own business. Successful by today's standards.

He spoke like Tony Robbins but more wise Grandpa, less salesman. The crowd clapped him off stage with tears and tithes. He was no sooner off stage than I realized he wasn't cool. He was addicted.

After swearing off the sauce, our speaker success story gained sixty pounds, took up smoking and presumably shuttled caffeine. This was the example on how to beat addiction.

What made this so much worse wasn't the fact that I noticed this, it was the fact that I noticed it so quickly. Like a quarterback taking all the credit for winning the big game, his behavior tainted his achievement. A guest speaker to my right whispered, "well, if that's alcohol free, give me a Corona."

Amen.

The comment reminded me of the sermon on the mount.

While our addicted friend was being judged by myself and others, we were forgetting to judge ourselves. "Why worry about a speck in your friend's eye when there's a log in yours."

Caffeine:

Over 90-percent of adult Americans consume caffeine every day. Over 30-percent of that number consumer 600mg or more. Some crazy caffeine cavaliers sip upwards of 6,000mg/day.

It's studied that 300mg of caffeine and below is safe, but that is rarely where we stop. In fact, that is about two cups of coffee.

It's not that caffeine is all bad, it's been shown to enhance mood, improve performance and increase metabolic turnover. However, when taken in excess, it does the opposite.

Caffeine is a stimulant. It down-regulates two sleep hormones. If we use it sparsely, no worries. The trouble begins when we continue to increase our dosage to feel the same high as when we first started consuming it.

The only option for the body is two up-regulate other sleep hormones, essentially, creating a negative loop feedback. Once we finally decide to leave Coffee in Columbia, we have two sleep hormones ultra high and two more on the rise. The difficult road back to "normal" is called withdrawal.

To avoid the addicted caffeine loop, keep it simple and sparse. Two cups a day and sleep more.

Birth Control:

Raise your hand if you take birth control.

Ok, raise your hand if you know birth control is a steroid.

Now, raise you hand the last time you condemned a profession athlete for taking steroids to hit a ball farther, while you were taking steroids to prevent life.

Hmmmmm … slap yourself with that hand.

About 30-percent of adult women in the US use oral birth control. The other small percentages use patches that contain mostly the same hormones that cease ovulation.

Many oral birth control pills, just like many oral performance enhancers, are 17 alpha-alkylated, meaning they contain a sort of poison meant to keep the liver busy while the real drug does its work.

I won't linger, but the hypocrisy is too much to go unnoticed. If ya really wanna keep screwing like rabbits with no consequences, how bout we have the man go under the knife, instead of the woman living under the pill?

Ibuprofen:
Sold generally under the brand name Advil, Ibuprofen is a drug classified as an NSAID, or non-steroidal anti-inflammatory drug. While it's true, some over the counter anti-pain med users exercise caution, as we should with any drug, many simply throw caution to the wind and pop pills like pez.

While the rare trip to the drugstore for post surgery relief or the worst migraine in the world may warrant pain modification, daily living doesn't. Food turns into addiction when it becomes an uncontrollable expression of poor behavior. Pain medication is no different.

Today, athletes celebrate the joys of "RIICE"- Rest, Ice, Ibuprofen, Compression, Elevation. The downside of this is of course is not only the addictive behavior, but the damage done.

Ibuprofen works as a COX inhibitor. Basically, it prevents Prostaglandins from working.

Certain experts would leave you to believe some Prostaglandins are harmful. when in truth, there are just unbalanced. Prostaglandins are either pro-inflammatory or anti-inflammatory. God didn't mess up, we need them both.

"Food turns into addiction when it becomes an uncontrollable expression of poor behavior. Pain medication is no different."

Ibu's, more or less, cut off the signal meant to heal damaged micro tears in muscles from overuse, training or whatever. While we think we are preventing pain, we are actually preventing recovery. Preventing recovery leads to injury.

The kind of everyday inflammation we experience is best explained as growing pains. Assuming you move like you have some sense then all that muscle soreness comes from two places, bad diet, or good activity. Slamming a daily dose of "Vitamin I" will not only prevent you from improving, it will make you worse.

In the future, exchange the Ibu's for fish oil or just stopping rubbing it and be a man.

Alcohol:
I watched my dad drink himself stupid everyday of my young life. His last painful years were mostly survived in a blue recliner with a motor. It stood up for him.

A lifestyle of excessive drinking and horrible eating gave him a stroke. The stroke gave him a lisp and a mind that didn't work so good. I loved my dad. I miss him.

I would've followed his path if it weren't for his example. God used my dad to show me how NOT to live, a gift I won't waste. That's why I'm writing this book ... for him. For you. For me.

Alcohol bypasses the stomach and works a lot like fructose. Interestingly, the two very substances the most dangerous to the human condition work the same way. Alcohol poisons the liver and it's surrounding tissue, while raising insulin levels and crashing several others systems in the body. Including, but not limited to:

Fat loss
Calcium retention
Growth hormone maintenance
Testosterone production
Depression, and more

Alcohol is an energy substrate and sort of works its way to the front line of the body. After all, it's poison and our bodies hate it. They can't burn it off quick enough.

Since alcohol is a sugar it is given preferential treatment before everything else. Meaning, all that gym hard work comes after that alcohol lazy ness. After all, you can't burn fat if your liver is busy cleaning your insides or burning sugar. And you can't pick on smokers or fast food eaters with a beer in your hand.

There is no safe amount of booze. There is only pain and suffering attached to a product, that for all intensive purposes, is legal poison. Buddhists abstain from it, so did John the baptist and God fearing Christians today. Not to mention the Spartans who remained on the wagon all their days. And if the Spartans did it, it has to be awesome.

Nicotine:

Nicotine works as a stimulant and is one of the few substances to cross the blood brain barrier. Nicotine has been compared to heroin and others illegal substances for its supremely addictive properties.

Tobacco is a night shade, making it not only addictive, but allergenic. Users experience the effects differently, but it's safe to say that there is no safe amount of the cash crop this country once held so dear.

⋏

At the end of our seminar, I went up to the walking chimney who had spoken about his ability to leave addiction at the curb

"Congratulations on your achievement," I said.

"Thanks a lot man. Have you overcome an addiction?," he asked.

"No, but my dad did. He was an alcoholic and he isn't anymore."

"That's great, how's he doing?"

"He's dead. He gave up the bottle and started smoking more. He loved donuts too."

CHAPTER 16

STOP SNACKING

Something is terribly wrong.

They're called jumping jacks but she's forgetting the "jacks" part. Her feet are moving, her face nearly as red as her shirt, but her arms are glued to her sides.

The path to her is crowded with athletes of all sorts, old, young, brave, scared, rookie veteran. She's not new, not experienced, and as far from the front of the class as possible.

"Pillars," I call, the next movement in the warm-up. And that's when I see it. A middle aged mother of three scared to death of jumping jacks, because they make her shirt come up and show her stomach.

I teach on.

"The fidget" I named it so many years ago, after seeing it happen hundreds of times, is when someone, unhappy with their body or outfit or both, can't stop pulling at the hem of their shirt. If it's not a disorder it should be, like biting your nails or picking your face or washing you hands too much.

Who cares, you say, *it's their body. Let them fidget all they want.*

That would be fine if ever errant tick didn't mean we weren't fully present. Because if you're thinking about your belly, you're missing something else. Something important.

"What's on your mind," I asked Deb in the back of class, hair done like she was heading down the runway next, nails painted flawlessly and make-up, somehow perfect after a workout.

"I swear--I know you've heard this before--but I've been following and nothing's happening," Deb said.

This is about the time I get all Sherlock Holmes on people. I read their face like fine print on an advertisement. Every action is an alarm clocks telling me more than they want. It didn't use to be this way, I used to take these types of cries as truth. Once, a time and two times ago, I gave everyone the benefit of the doubt. But dieters lie more than criminals, gamblers and alcoholics combined.

I searched for her tell, I looked for the grand canyon in her story, I stared as if she may burst into a succubus at any moment. Nothing. I believed her. Or rather, I believe that she really believed what she was telling me.

We started to leave the workout floor, her husband who was her partner that day gave me that "please God, do something look." I nodded and closed the door to my office.

"Humor me and write down your meals for the last three days," I said.

"Ok, but I promise, everything is Paleo."

"I don't doubt you, but I have to find the problem."

Her mind surprised me the way a two-year surprises a parent the first time they swear. She had exactly the same meal three times a day. She wasn't a small girl, but the meals were. She guaranteed it had been exactly like this for week … so had she.

Diets are math problems. What do I need to add, what can I subtract? Puzzled, I searched for the solution.

"This is everything you put in your mouth?," I asked more rhetorically than anything.

"Well, not everything," she said. "Those are meals, I don't count the snacks because they're so small and still Paleo."

Relief, like narrowly missing a four car pile up, set-in.

"Tell me a little more about these snacks," I said.

"Whenever I'm hungry, I get a handful of mixed nuts."

"And how often are you hungry?"

"I'm not sure but it can't be too much."

"Ok, how often do you buy these snacks at the store?"

"We go to the store twice a week and I usually get three jars."

A small jar of nuts, if it really is the small one, is about 8-ounces and 1,500 Calories. She was snacking on this every day, it was very paleo and very much halting her progress.

"I only eat a handful or so when I need it," she said interrupting my silent calculation.

"It sounds like you need it enough to finish a jar a day," I said.

⋏

I'm not saying the occasional snack will derail your plans, nor am I saying avoid those 300 calories of nuts until you almost gnaw your arm off and order a pizza. I'm saying that even healthy snacks add up to unhealthy results.

Four Snacking Killers

Insulin:
Everything we eat potentially releases insulin. And, more importantly, when we are in a fed state, we stop burning fat.

Stopping a meal short of satisfaction only to snack soon after means you're burning less and less fat while eating healthy food. What do you wanna be better at … storing fat or burning fat?

Discipline:
The constant need to eat paleo snack after paleo snack is crude self-therapy preventing us from dealing with deeper issues. Hiding behind food, even paleo food, is a spiral that will end badly. Keep you hands off desk candy, brunch specials and numerous paleo picnics. Carry a bottle of water and every time you would snack … sip.

Leptin:

Leptin is seriously important hormone produced oddly enough from our fat cells. But just as we can become resistant to insulin, we can become resistant to Leptin. And the fatter you are, the more resistant you are, the more resistant you are, the more hungry you feel.

To ensure proper leptin levels; eat fat. Instead of 50-percent of your calories from protein, some from fat and some from carbs. Ensure that at least 50-percent of your daily caloric intake comes from fat, followed by 20-percent protein or so.

WKO fasted:

That little pre-workout "I'm a runner from the mid-nineties and I need to carb load" meal you're still pounding prior to a workout is ensuring you won't be burning anything during your workout. Workout fasted whenever possible.

If you truly feel like you have to snack, then start eating more at each meal and watch the fat burning kick back in.

Two weeks after my talk and Deb was down six pounds. She said she ate nuts with her meals, not in between them, but didn't really lessen her food intake.

Calories in vs Calories out … not always.

CHAPTER 17

MULTIPLE MEALS SUCK

"**I didn't think** I was going to make it through the drive-through," Mike said.

"Why didn't you go in?," I asked.

"Because, I thought I'd pass out. I was sweating and breathing hard and feeling heavy and getting weak all at the same time. When I finally got to the window, I ordered two large milk shakes. I took the top off one and slammed it before I even left the window. I drank the second one as I was pulling out of the parking lot. I drove back into the drive-thru and got another one. Then I started to feel better."

At the time, all I wanted was Mike's muscles. He was injecting insulin everyday and getting bigger by the second. He wasn't as big as some of the superheroes I dreamt of, but he was close.

Somehow, during Mike's offseason, I missed his dramatic fat gain and appearance. His face was round like a basketball and red. All the lines that once shaped every muscle he had we're blurred or gone, a balloon that would deflate if you pricked it.

Mike was an idiot.

He became my case study for real world insulin injections coupled with stupidity. Today, we call Mike's behavior, "The Standard American Diet." The difference is, Mike used a syringe, Americans use doughnuts.

Natural Play Time

When Mike entered a room everyone knew. His biceps blocked out the sun, he wore tank tops in the winter time, sunglasses at night, nicest guy in the world but not too bright. I wanted his muscles but insulin scared me. Instead of injections, I turned to the next best thing; sugar.

I studied numerous articles and medical texts before I finally came to a post workout concoction meant to spike blood glucose, thereby raising insulin. Insulin, after all, is the one of the most anabolic substances in the body.

My post workout meal began with milk, as dairy is more insulinogenic than white bread. The simple combination of casein protein, galactose, and amino acid profile, combined with its IGF (insulin growth factor) stimulation, bovine insulin, and various other hormones make it a powerful candidate for the insulin surge I was looking for.

I added Glutamine next. Glutamine is a glycogenic amino acid, meaning, it can turn to sugar. Especially when you ingest 70 grams of it at a time.

Glycerol, the next ingredient, added staying power. This thickener is used in protein bars and is essentially a sugar bond.

Dextrose was added to the tune of 100 grams. Equivalent to 400 grams of carbohydrates from pure blood glucose. This is the stuff they put in Gatorade and sell to kids.

Immediately after a workout, I blended all this together and chugged the sweet concoction. About fifteen minutes later, I passed out.

Within six short weeks, I was 25 lb. heavier and all I did was add this shake. I gained fat, lots of fat.

Thankfully, I was a hair smarter than, Mike. Insulin is by far one of the most powerful hormones in our bodies. Until we respect it, until we fear it, it literally eats us alive.

Insulin Primer

Insulin is a hormone produced in the pancreas. Insulin is generally released by healthy individuals in response to eating carbohydrates which are broken down to single molecules for digestion called monosaccharides.

When these monosaccharides are digested in the lining of the small intestine, they become glucose. Glucose can be used immediately, or it can be converted to glycogen and stored in the muscle walls and liver.

Liver glycogen is generally full after the first meal of the day. Our liver holds nearly 50 grams of carbohydrates at any one time.

Liver glycogen can feed brain and red blood cells and other organs, but it's a poor substitute for fat fed organs like the heart and kidneys.

Muscle glycogen amounts to 3-percent or so of the muscle weight, and cannot be sent to other parts of the body. It feeds the muscle and only the muscle.

Once the liver has converted glucose to glycogen, it can convert it back when needed for immediate energy. This process is called glycogenolysis. However, muscles aren't so friendly. They cannot convert glycogen to glucose. Muscle glycogen is converted to pyruvic acid and then converted to ATP (adenosine tri-phosphate) in a process called glycolysis.

Insulin ensures glucose, the most toxic compound in our body, doesn't last for any longer than necessary. Insulin is released when excessive amounts of glucose, not dedicated to the liver or muscles, remain the blood.

Insulin comes along and mops up the unnecessary glucose and shuttles this nutrient into fat cells for use as fuel later. At least this is what happens to a well functioning human.

A type I diabetic has a dysfunction which doesn't allow them to produce their own insulin and they must take it via injection.

A type II diabetic produces insulin, but has become resistant to the effects. The high level of toxic blood glucose remains in the blood and hyperglycemia sets in, including a malady of other disorders. Insulin resistance is usually created by eating "The Standard American Diet" of high carbs, low fat, and low quality protein.

The cells in a type II diabetic resist the energy the insulin is carrying and trying to store within them. Therefore, the body produces more insulin until the pancreas, which actually devotes very little effort to insulin production, cannot keep up.

Basically, insulin is storing excess energy and making fat in the time of feast, preparing for a time of famine.

Eating fewer meals and eating fewer carbs
Carbohydrates are not essential to our diet.

When we give up carbs long enough, we become ketotic. Depending on who you are, this metabolic shift can be uncomfortable and misdiagnosed.

For instance. My fasting blood glucose is generally under 70 mg/dl. ADA's Recommended blood glucose is 90 mg/dl. As you can see, hypoglycemia is purely reactive. What feels good for me may feel horrible for someone else.

Someone ingesting 400 grams of carbohydrates a day, will not experience low blood sugar when they eliminate 90-percent of their daily carbohydrate intake, they'll get withdrawal. Alcoholics and junkies know this, the obese call it hypoglycemia and eat more sugar.

Alcoholics don't wean off the bottle, they quit drinking or they never beat the addiction.

Fasting Blood Glucose/Hemoglobin a1c

We can decide our quality, and relative longevity of life, if we control our blood glucose levels. The less sugar the better.

FBG is the pin prick thing that you pick up at the store for $30. Measure fasted, one hour postprandial, and two hours postprandial. We're looking for a fasted measurement under 80 mg/dl, and postprandial of no more than 140 mg/dl.

Side note: FBG can be elevated in low carb eaters. Esterified fatty acids and glycerol molecules from ketosis and triglyceride breakdown, make the reading a little wonky.

Ha1c is a measure of sticky sugar attached to your red-blood cells which die off every three months or so. This measure is more accurate when it comes to sugar. Ha1c shows a timeline, not just a day in time. We are looking for 5 mg/dl or under.

By the year 2050, over thirty-one-million Americans will be over 80-years-old. Some studies say half of those folks will have Alzheimer's. Another 10-percent will have Parkinson's.

Dr. Theodore B. VanItallie, had Parkinson's sufferers ingest; 90% fat/ 8% protein/ and 2% carbs." Almost all symptoms stopped.

Dr. Theo, was trying to help people lose weight. In the process, he stumbled on "Hyper-ketosis." In Dr Theo's experiments, less sugar meant less insulin. Weight loss followed, so did other symptoms not previously thought to be sugar related.

Insulin ensures excess glucose doesn't hang out in our bloodstream. When there is more glucose than necessary, it's like battery acid leaking out of the battery.

Post myopic means can't regenerate. This is what happens to certain cells after too much sugar for too long. For a while, neuroplasticity takes over and cells connections change routes. However, after all the routes are gummed up with traffic, information loses its path. In fact, that's why it's called aging.

AGE's= Advanced Glycated End-products

Through a cross linking process, better explained by a chemist, AGE's mount an attack leaving our eyes, brain, skin, and everything else in between worse for wear.

The Warburg Effect

Dr. Warburg, a scientist from the depression, thought it would be cool to prevent disease as opposed to treat it. He called it, "nutritional prevention", or "nutritional insurance."

Genotyping means "born to." Some call it pre-disposed. The opposite end lies phenotyping. Phenotyping is what we create ourselves to be.

Take, for instance, alcoholism: Supposedly, the child from an alcoholic is 60-percent more likely to become addicted themselves. Children of drunks are genotyped to be drunks. Whether I believe that or not is irrelevant. What is relevant is the fact that even if that were true, one must still activate the gene. Whether you are more likely to be a drunk or not, you still have to chose to drink to become one.

Dr. Warburg noticed that most tumors and cancers were fed by glucose. Before medication was all the rage, Warburg thought, if sugar is the fuel, stop eating sugar. It worked.

Later that year, Dr. Warburg won the Nobel Peace Prize for his ketogenic diet research.

But, eating a low-carb diet isn't profitable. I have no clue what became of the good Doctor.

Why multiple meals suck

Insulin is just a storage hormone, glucagon is just the opposite. Whenever there is no carbohydrates present, glucagon has the ability to kick in and release the energy stored in fat.

Personally, back in my immature diet days, I regularly consumed seven meals a day. Incorrectly, I was under the belief that smaller meals "stoked the metabolism," even though human biology clearly does not support this. I ate every two hours for years, while forcing my athletes to do the same.

The tools I picked up from the bodybuilder trade hypnotized me into believing their way was the only way. Thankfully, my allegiance to douchebag magazines full of advertisements gave way to my "there has to be a better way" mind. It's not that you can't make it work, it's that it's nowhere near the simplest or healthiest way.

Multiple meals fell into the fitness limelight because the food pyramid recommends a high carb diet. Carbohydrates don't satisfy hunger, they increase blood sugar which we constantly regulate with more food.

Blood sugar is radically elevated for two hours or so after a meal heavy in carbohydrates. Hormonal changes combined with rising insulin wreaks havoc. About two or three hours after that, our hormones cascade back down as does our blood sugar. Withdrawal.

Multiple meals, for most of us, are treatment not cure.

Muscley Mike and the Bottom Line

To eliminate the need for frequent feedings; eat fat!

I didn't figure this out until long after I severed my relationship with Mike and his friends who were willing to do anything in the name of muscle. What's odd, isn't the fact that Mike shot insulin to get huge, it's that he wasn't doing anything different than the droves of humans stuffing a million sugary Calories down their throats everyday.

Mike used a syringe and worked out, others use a doughnut and don't get off the couch. When it comes to risky, what's the difference?

CHAPTER 18

CROSSFIT: THE CURE TO EXERCISE

It began at eight-o-clock every morning and it lasted about an hour.

My boss, his wife and me, scrunched inside a shoebox of an office talking business. When I was just starting out it was cool, a barely 20-something trainer talking about the gym. You'd be surprised how fast cool wears off when you discover that your dreams don't exactly line-up with your path.

All we did was talk business. Not training. Not workout design. Not diet. Not the best way to keep people on track and getting results, but business. Billing problems, contracts, cleaning, how to get the most people to sign on the dotted line and never actually use the gym.

I was a part time trainer, full time gym manager, and I hated it. Business, a necessary evil, doesn't belong in the fitness world. Yes, you have to pay your bills, and yes you need a system to deal with the details, but hour long, daily meetings about turning people into dollar signs is not what I signed up for.

So I quit.

Not outright, I didn't have the balls for that, so I stepped down as manager and began personal training for a living.

Still, something was missing. There's not enough hours in the day and my methods, while they worked, we're boring and esoteric at best. It wasn't so much getting my athletes to fall in love with training as much as it was getting them to fall for me. If I wasn't there, they didn't care to train.

Every night I studied and everyday, when I wasn't training athletes, I was drawing diagrams, imagining ways to make fitness fun, dreaming. In between that I was suffering, practicing what I preached with dry chicken breasts and broccoli, bicep curls and hours on the treadmill.

There had to be something better.

CrossFit, the cure to exercise:
Since my best friend turned me onto a gritty website more than eight years ago, I've coached CrossFit. They say you only move twice? That's what it felt like. Even though I'd never heard or attempted anything CrossFit, it felt like I was going home, to a place full of familiar aromas and automatic emotions. I never looked back.

Gone were the treadmills, the bicep curls and tricep extensions, the hour long workouts and three hours of cardio when I needed to look really good. Most importantly, gone was the boredom. I always loved how I felt after training, that's why I never stopped, but much of the time I hated doing it. Not CrossFit. Even when it's something you've done before, it feels new. Familiar but welcomed .. except running. Screw that.

When I told my good friend, who also happened to be my boss, I wanted to open an affiliate, I expected him to be happy for me. We had no clue what CrossFit really was all those years ago, this was before Games and just after Youtube. I expected his support, hell, maybe he'll want to be my partner.

He fired me the next day.

Have you ever been rear ended when you were watching the road in front of you? That's what it felt like, all eyes on the prize, following all the rules and trying to make a life for myself. WHAM, some jackass plows into my new car and now I have whiplash.

The next few months were hard. No gym would let me workout for fear of competition. Banks weren't offering money and my athletes were going elsewhere.

CrossFit kept me going.

I watched clip after clip, studied everything in The CrossFit Journal and believed like I never had before. CrossFit is the way, and no matter what, I can teach it to people.

My blind obsession paid off. We were approved for a loan and Practice CrossFit opened in Troy, Ohio in 2007. And even after all my studying, I thought CrossFit was too good to be true. I still trained three hours a day and worked every single muscle group, including my forearms and neck, individually. For cardio, sure, CrossFit was king, but for all out strength, for the ultra low body fat I was used to, I needed long bouts on steppers isolation training.

Right?

That first loan bought barbells, plates and rubber matting, all CrossFit friendly gear. It also bought a leg press, leg extension, leg curl and lat pull-down. The CrossFitter in me screaming to get out knew I was being stubborn, a pastor coming to terms with the fact that he'd been preaching the wrong sermon his entire life. It's not that exercise is bad, it's certainly better than lazy, but CrossFit wasn't exercise. It was training. Even if you had no hopes of the stage or field of dreams, better at CrossFit becomes your goal, and better at CrossFit meant more fit. Exercise is just activity.

In 2007, two months after I opened my first affiliate, I finally went all in with CrossFit. We sold all that waste of space equipment for pennies on the dollar and bought more bumpers. It wasn't that the old ways of isolation exercises and duration cardio didn't serve a purpose, it's that CrossFit, in less than a third of the time, offered so much more than all show and no go. With CrossFit, I looked better, got stronger and felt like an athlete, something, that as a bodybuilder, no matter how good I looked, I never felt before.

Community:
Passion was all that saved us those first rocky months. Convincing my one-on-one athletes that CrossFit was the way, and everything we'd done before more or less a waste, challenging. Like me they fought.

"So you won't be training me anymore?"

"So we don't need to get on the treadmill?"

"So a 10-minute workout is enough?"

With science I did my best to calm their fears. That's like fighting an Army with pebbles. No one cares about science when they think their ass is about to grow or their personal time is about to be invaded. Hell, even I was unsure of what it was going to be like. Instead of me and one athlete at a time, it would be me and whoever showed up to workout at anytime. Training turned from selling myself and personality, to selling CrossFit. Luckily, CrossFit results are addicting and passion is contagious.

Most stayed, if nothing else for the novelty, to see how this whole CrossFit thing would crash and burn. I mean--flipping tires along main street, running in the rain and pull-ups until your hands bled--how can that last?

Naturally, like a canyon formed from a creek, a community developed.

At first I didn't notice, how close we'd all become through workouts. How we did our best to train together and how we started to genuinely want the best results for those we trained with. It was so very different than everything I remembered about working out. CrossFit, unlike exercise, was like being on a team. Like belonging.

Back then the CrossFit community was building and the distance between affiliates and lag in media meant your own little slice of heaven was all yours. Over the years, as the landscape changed and we added boxes by the dozens, everyone realized that it wasn't thrusters growing this thing, it was people. A community forming through effort, backed by science, full of strangers who became the best of friends.

CrossFit is constantly varied functional movement at the utmost intensity. And when that formula permeates through athletes all over the globe, creating an undeniable connection, a powerful tribe rises like a Phoenix from ashes long forgotten. That's what makes CrossFit endearing to so many and why CrossFit endures and always will. Not exercise, but training. Not a crowd, but a community.

CHAPTER 19

Living Everyday Paleo

I've saved a handful of special emails over the years. This is one of them.

"Dear, Josh

I wanted to say thank you for everything. My husband, Joe, met you at a seminar and something you said finally stuck. He returned home from your speech renewed. He has spent his entire adult life overweight. In fact, his entire life. I'm no prize either but his weight problem was severe and always left him with a very poor self image.

My husband tried every fad diet and exercise program around. We have together spent thousands on gym memberships. We failed to use those membership two weeks after we purchased them. Our home is full of equipment that takes up room until it makes it's way to Ebay, or Craigslist, or a garage sale. Together we failed miserably every time. For me I move on and make excuses to feel better.

A friend invited my husband to go hear you speak locally. He was skeptical but his friends winning argument was a description of your personality. Joe attended your seminar over eight months ago and has since elevated his weight loss goal to 85 lb. He now wears size 34 jeans. He plays softball in a league and smiles a lot. He wants to go out with our friends. He is a different man. A man I knew was there. Now, he is a stranger to everyone else but me. Thank you for this.

While I am grateful for what you have taught him through your articles, I'm looking for your help also. I am now the "fat" one in the relationship. Before I was the skinny one of the group trying to help him out. Every time we made a fitness commitment in the past, he always failed before me. I simply attributed my failure to his because his was first. In my mind, he had to be the weak one.

Once he failed I had to quit because I didn't want him to feel worse. But now I continue to realize I wasn't happy either, I just was focused on him and his goals. Now he's focused on me and I keep failing.

First, I didn't believe in the Paleo diet when he started. I was only supportive because I thought Joe would fail. Months later and pounds lighter, I am a firm Paleo believer. But I'm confused.

What I don't understand, and why I think I'm failing, is all these different versions of Paleo. All the different approaches. Josh, how do you eat Paleo in everyday normal life? How can one Paleo cookbook advise one thing and another give the exact opposite advice? How can a rookie like me make the right decisions with so much conflicting data? Josh, how can I be successful like my husband when we are two different people?

He eats the same thing everyday, but I need variety. He eats what you call Paleo, then when I sit at the table thinking I'm doing good he says, "that's not Paleo." After he tells me that all I want is a chocolate cake.

Josh, I love my husband, but his success is somehow hurting me, or at least making me see what I was missing. Can you please help me?"

Everyday Paleo

In the beginning, many of us find Paleo living inconvenient. Prepared meat or veggies are cumbersome for folks immediately switching from the drive through side of life.

We can survive and thrive on everyday Paleo early on by making changes that look a lot more like experiments than rituals. Somewhere a Paleo fanatic is turning in his grave and that's fine. We're not looking to fit any definition other than "Do only what heals, nothing that hurts."

If it fits that, it's Paleo.

Best to become a Paleo Poser as opposed to a fanatic. Posers have the freedom of experiment. You won't go to neolithic hell if you use silverware, turn on fluorescent lights, or cook with an oven. Paleo Posers accept Paleo as a name and helpful tool, not a shelter to make them elite or better than someone else

Quick tricks of the trade

- Fast food trips are not perfect, but if they get you through the day avoiding bread and candy - awesome. You will learn to plan better but emergencies happen, and there is always an option.
- Deli meat is like fast food. It contains very un-paleo preservatives, but it's better than many alternatives and sometimes eating better requires more of a babyish step than outlandish leap. Eating the occasional piece of deli meat is better than shunning all the teachings because you're missing one commandment.
- While we are talking about it; perfect is the enemy.
- Perfect becomes an excuse to fail. Continue to increase your paleo utility belt by disregarding perfection. Continued improvement, while not as good as your neighbor, is far better than failure.
- Nuts are a solution to problems that haven't yet shown up. I don't recommend snacking but when hunger calls early, better to eat

something approved right away then mistakenly rely on willpower that may fail and lead you to pizza.

- Jerky and dehydrated meat is still meat ... kinda. If you make this an exception rarely instead of frequently it most likely will have no negative effects.
- Make friends in the restaurant business. In my hometown I have three go to restaurants that use coconut oil. I send them business and they provide me an alternative to cooking.
- Bacon isn't the best option, but it feels like cheating.
- When you're at your table, eat big and fill up on fat. That way, when you're in a pinch, you will be more likely to sustain good habits.

Whats up with all the different versions; Paleo, pseudo-paleo, primal, caveman....

Today everyone is an expert. Everyone an evangelist of their denomination. What to do?

On the surface there is no simple answer; they all make a convincing argument. But when you learn to read between the lines some things stand out.

1. Using the word "I"

Mark's Daily Apple, the world's voice to the primal way of life says "I" often.

He is of course referring to his personal actions. The guy helps a lot of people and we should celebrate him for that. But he is also making a bigger buck with a bigger casting net by phrases like; *Personally, cheese doesn't affect me, but if it hurts you, eliminate it.*

While I advocate a lot of what the dude says this sounds a lot like justification. Mark Sisson himself seems to want these cravings and he seems to want others to accept his stance. Therefore, he makes an argument for them and then poses it as something you can decide whether or not is right for you, after all, it works for him.

Whenever I utilized variety days (cheating), I would have McDonalds and pizza and sometimes ice cream. No matter how many arguments I had for it, and no matter how much I wanted it, it just doesn't work for me or anyone - ever.

I would gain eight-pounds of water, my FBG would go up and I would feel like death. Not to mention the fact that weekly cheating is nothing more than addiction suppression. If we are willing to justify one thing, we are willing to justify everything. I know, I have done this my whole life.

2. Making others feel silly

This trick is generally used by the academics. For some reason they think their Paleo is better than the street performers Paleo because they have pretty letters behind their name.

The whole time folks like this speak louder and louder folks like us get farther and farther away from the noise. I'm more than happy trying every road to success, never being wetted to one theory or dogma. My way is a whole bunch of experiments put together and I would change it on a dime if something better came along. I don't need a degree to tell me if I feel and look sick.

3. Recipes for disaster

Everyone has a Paleo cookbook now, everyone is a Paleo Chef. Almost everyone claims their "almost paleo" is the way to go for you and yours. Almost everyone is learning to make a buck by manipulating others. Simply eat; meat, nuts, seeds, vegetables, no starch, no sugar, no alcohol.

Cookbooks look pretty on the table and come in handy for 2% of the people that buy them. The rest of us just won't prioritize the time to make those recipes happen. In fact, some recipes that claim to be paleo we really shouldn't eat anyway.

Paleo cookbooks sell lifestyles.

They put some awesome photo of some tempting dish on the cover that you'd be lucky to make once. Looking at them sends our brains into pleasure mode by releasing dopamine. Dopamine is strongly related to food and sex. A cookbook is food porn.

Also, when we see those fancy dishes on the cover we think of the folks we can entertain and have compliment our culinary arts. We think of the feeling we know we can make others have by having them enjoy the dish we can make for them.

Just remember this the next time you're intoxicated by a book with little knowledge and photoshopped pics; There is no substitute for chicken and the world hasn't seen a new vegetable for a long time. Ask yourself, what is a cookbook going to teach me that I don't already know?

The green-eyed-monster

Amy's husband dropped 30 lb. I imagine he turned the head of a female or two, and I bet he spoke with renewed confidence.

Amy felt threatened by his success, not intimidated by meat and vegetables. It took her a bit to admit that, but after she did she settled in and starting eating until her heart was content, while following one simple rule. The only Paleo rule we have …

Do only what heals and nothing that hurts.

She's 42 lb. lighter as I write this.

CHAPTER 20

LOOKING HEALTHY ISN'T ALWAYS BEING HEALTHY

Our shirts hit the floor at the same time, five reps into the workout, surrounding us like sweaty casualties of a war sponsored by Rogue.

"Time," I screamed well before Doug.

After I collapsed I watched Doug keep fighting. He was new to CrossFit but you wouldn't know it by his physique.

He was just over six-feet tall, shoulders like melons sitting below mountainous slabs of sinew and muscle called traps. His arms weren't huge, more agile and defined--Spartan, something you'd see in greek art that men want and women love.

Like the sister Doug was visiting, he was naturally lean. I hate guys like that. The ones who do whatever the hell they want while I get fat drinking water.

"Time," Doug said well after me.

Spent, sweating and shirtless he hit the ground. The crowd watching us came in for fist bumps.

"What do you eat?," I asked.

"Nothing particular," he said. "I usually eat when I'm hungry and try to not eat junk food. I guess I don't really have a particular diet."

I was expecting that. In fact, his sister, lifetime athlete and CrossFit Games competitor, has the same body type, built like an actress working around the clock to get the part of Amazon Princess, or Supergirl.

Even the women who say they would never like to have that much muscle lie when they stare down her beauty. The correct statement is, "I don't wanna work that hard."

Doug and his sister were proof positive; looking healthy doesn't always mean being healthy.

Pheno vs Geno

Not long ago, scientists believed hundreds of thousands of separate Genes go into making this little thing we call human. That myth was eventually squashed and today we are sure it's between 20,000-25,000.

That's still a lot of genes to play with. Cancer, Alcoholism, Dwarfism, Blindness, Fatness; there's a gene for everything.

Stem Cells, Your Surroundings, Your Friends

Have you ever noticed insurance agents are religiously fat? Can you think of another habitually out of shape profession? Computer programmers, desk jockeys, preachers; bakers perhaps? It's true, not all of them are but you get the point. The questions is, would anyone given one of those environments take on the trait of the majority? Or, did they give a pre-existing condition an environment to grow?

Phenotyping is like a human stem cell complete with shoes and an attitude. Stick one skinny stem cell beside enough fat cells and whala, that blank cell turns fat like the rest.

Heredity states that I should be a rampant alcoholic because my dad was one. In fact, there is a 70-percent chance that I am a drunk waiting to happen. However, one critical thing must happen first; I have to drink.

Kids from the hood have ventured to Harvard. Orphans from the gutter have become world class physicians. Children of drunks have died without a drop of the sauce in their soul.

Survival of the fittest rears it's head at the most opportune time. The fittest in today's society need not run the fastest or be the strongest to prevent other competition from stealing their food or mate. Today, the barrier between those naturally selected for demise is little more than willpower. It's avoiding the genetics we were all born with.

Paleo man didn't have to diet from his favorite sweets or packaged goodies, the dude didn't have the temptation. Regardless if he had the gene, he didn't have the light switch.

"Heredity states that I should be a rampant alcoholic because my dad was one. In fact, there is a 70-percent chance that I am a drunk waiting to happen. However, one critical thing must happen first. I have to drink."

The fittest on the planet have all the cancer causing, body deforming genes like the rest of us. The fittest often just say no. Never have humans had it so easy to be so fit and never have we been more sick. Today's predator is the media. Today's prey is us.

Genotyping

Around five-percent of the population will be born with something terminal.

Genotyping means potential and likelihood, whereas Phenotyping means desire and action. Most of the time, it's our actions that condemn, not birth.

For instance, fat people make other fat people more fat. If your main goal is to rid yourself of 50, 40, 30, or 20 lb. of extra weight, it's going to be hard to do with anyone beside you comfortable with gaining it.

"Never have humans had it so easy to be so fit and never have we been more sick."

Detaching yourself from fat people is one way to get thin, but while this tactic may definitely cause you to eat less by association, or lack thereof, it won't solve the reason for the eating in the first place. More than likely, food was your medication suppressing something deep seeded within you.

If you are habitually surrounded by complaining, more than likely that's what you will do. If all you are is drained by others, chances are you will suck on whatever gives you their neck. Seven desserts at a table full of plus sizes may be your tipping point. One of the easiest ways to avoid getting hit, is never starting a fight.

Metabolically Obese.

On the outside Doug was a novel everyone wanted to get lost in. Inside he was more tawdry-tale than bestseller.

Metabolically Obese is the term coined for folks who look like a 20-something sex god on the outside, full of strength, speed and confidence. Internally, however, they look like a heart attack waiting to happen.

Doug was willing to do whatever required to be a better athlete, not necessarily a healthier one ... not yet anyway.

Doug's Biomarkers when we started:

HDL-39
LDL-124
H1Ac-5.7
C-Reactive Protein-1.9
Triglycerides 212
Body Fat-11%

Now, these numbers won't put you in a grave tomorrow, but everyone one of them, except the ultra low body-fat, demonstrates metabolic syndrome.

Metabolic syndrome or "Syndrome X" was first thought to be caused by obesity. After we get fat, the theory states, a cascade of disorders follow. However, "Syndrome X's" founder, Dr. Kaplan, discovered getting fat was one of the side effects, not the cause.

Kaplan discovered that first we become insulin resistant due the repeated ingestion of too many carbohydrates. Then our good cholesterol becomes bad, or bad cholesterol becomes worse. Fasting blood glucose begins to resemble a diabetic and we live in constant inflammation.

As I mentioned earlier, Doug ate whatever the commercials and supplement ads told him he should. Everyday Calories like breads and pastas and yogurts. Foods that would leave the rest of us just as fat on the outside, as well as the inside.

But Doug wasn't fat, nor was his sister no matter the menu. Fat simply wasn't a side-effect for them.

Six months after Doug and I's first conversation, and diet reformation, we rematched.

Shirtless again, we stayed beside one another, barbell in hand. He didn't look different, but that didn't matter three minutes in when I needed to breath and he kept moving.

"Time," he called first.

After we recovered, I congratulated Doug for stomping me into the ground, he opened his cooler and removed his post-workout meal.

"What's in the cooler?," I asked.

"What you told me to eat," he said.

Four months later Doug's test results came back;

HDL-68
LDL-93
H1Ac-4.67
C-Reactive Protein-.9
Triglycerides 112
Body Fat-9%

Here's what Doug had to say:

"In March, 2009, I was in my final year of college. I went to the gym two or three times a week, I got seven hours of sleep a night. I ate what you're "supposed" to eat. I thought I was developing narcolepsy, one minute I would be sitting in class taking notes and the next I'd wake up drooling on my desk.

Everything changed for me later that month when I visited my sister. She introduced me to CrossFit and Josh and he explained the need for a few simple changes. Mainly, stop eating what you're "supposed" to eat. Initially I was skeptical. He wants me to get leaner by eating MORE food? But who was I to argue?

I cut the whole wheat. I cut Gatorade. I cut the heavy carbs before training. I felt better instantly."

ᴧ

Doug's results are typical. That is, of course, if we stop eating what we're suppose to eat.

CHAPTER 21

The Day I Almost Died

I was 24-years-old the day I almost died.

The sound of rush hour came through the open window with Virginia humidity. Good Morning America played on the TV. I remember thinking, *I'm going to die watching a talk show.*

The coach I was sitting on felt like Cool Whip, the way it let you sink and fade into nothing. The big bay window was perfect for watching tall Sycamores sway in the distance, from the kind of apartment yuppies pay too much for; in a town located in the middle of nowhere, with a population of far too many for my taste. The sort of town that had to be built up and not out.

My girlfriend at the time was talking to her roommate.

"But you can't seriously think she's attractive," my girlfriend said to her roommate about something meaningless on TV. "Josh, do you think she's pretty?," my girlfriend turned the argument towards me. Yeah I know this alone is an aneurysm waiting to happen, I see the trap.

"Well", I said, "I thinksg tjks if shan....."

"What?" my girlfriend said confused.

"Nothing," I managed to get out.

Hmmmm, that was weird, I thought. *I must be sleepy. And I must have dozed off on my arm because it feels weird.*

About three minutes later I perked up when I saw an advertisement on TV for skydiving.

"I habe alveys wntd," I said. What I meant to say was, "I have always wanted to do that."

Now I was freaking out. I gave my girlfriend a very odd look I'd never given her before - fear. She read it instantly.

I was slouching to the left and thought I'd been leaning on that arm, but when I looked, I realized I hadn't. It was propped nicely up on my leg. I touched it, nothing.

"I can't feel my left arm," I said. It didn't sound that way.

Touching a part of your body that doesn't respond to its owner is the dirtiest, most foreign feeling, like being raped in a dream.

My girlfriend's eyes grew and her nearly ginger skin flushed. Usually, she shrugged off everything. Not this time. I would have actually appreciated her concern if I didn't think I was dying. At least her roommate had answered a phone call just minutes ago, and we were alone.

She bolted off the couch as I stumbled to my feet. Her to a phone, me to a doorway. I had to test something. I placed my left arm in a door jam outside of her gaze. As she started to dial her mother, who happened to be a nurse, I slowly creaked open the door to our bedroom, took a big breath and put my hand in it. I slammed the door on my hand as hard as I could, three times.

I wept.

Not because it hurt, because it didn't. I cried because I was 24, half the age of my stroke-victim father, and I thought I'd become him.

He had described to me exactly how his stroke felt. The disconnect of brain and body. The ability to see what you want to say like a marquee on the street, but the inability to say it correctly. The loss of feeling, the haunting thoughts of a coffin, a wheelchair, a caregiver, all set in.

I continued my ramblings as my girlfriend described my symptoms to her mother.

I Prayed. "God, please don't let me be like my dad."

On the day I almost died, I bargained for my life like a car salesman. Reasoning, pleading with the God I continue to take for granted. "I work out. I go to church. I eat well...kinda. I don't deserve this."

"Not because it hurt, because it didn't. I cried because I was 24, half the age of my stroke-victim father, and I thought I'd just become him."

Can you fathom the moment you are hit with your mortality? Maybe it's happened to you, maybe it hasn't. Maybe you think, as I once did, you're Superman, and all the time in the world is yours.

Or maybe you argue fate. Weak people say that. They claim everything happens for a reason they are not assured of so it lessen their fear of death. I know, I did this for a long time - it's called fatalism.

Fate is for Fakers

Truly anticipating that death will come tomorrow, or the day after that, or the day after that makes you anxious for life the way it ought to be lived. We become eager to view each moment as its own blessing.

The day I realized just how weak and frail and horribly vulnerable I am, is the day I was given the biggest gift I ever received: Mortality.

Philosopher, Heidegger, called it, "Freedom towards death,"

"If I take death into my life, acknowledge it, and face it squarely, I will free myself from the anxiety of death and the pettiness of life - and only then will I be free to become myself," he said.

It's not a death wish, it's responsibility for our failure. It's living socially and changing the world, not having a social life which is just a diversion making us forget we are broken, damaged, and dying.

As Tyler Durden taught me, "First you have to give up. First you have to know, not fear, know, that one day you are going to die." Until you realize that, you will be imprisoned by fate, in a world where you believe your responsibility is nil, that everything is settled for you.

The day I came to terms with my own vulnerability has left me with many dark nights. They make me anxious for being better, like there is never enough time to help, to learn, to instruct, to create. The day I almost died is the day I began living.

Ten minutes after slamming my hand in a big oak door, I gave up. I think it's called acceptance.

Have you ever watched the ceiling above your bed rise, like the room's getting bigger, like you're disappearing, like the world is forgetting you?

My girlfriend was checking my pulse. I looked at her to save me. I have never wanted anyone to help me before, much less save me. For the first time, I cried in front of her.

"The day I realized just how weak and frail and horribly vulnerable I am, is the day I was given the biggest gift I ever received: Mortality."

The thoughts of my father walking with a cane and slurring crept into my head. I felt like I'd been leading troops to war and I'd led them straight into an ambush. Most of all, I felt guilty for the way I treated my dad.

I was so impatient with him. "How can he know what to say but not be able to say it."

I cried for my dad. I cried because I took everyday for granted and thought he should just get better.

I'm sorry I was so weak, dad. I wish you could've read this. I wish I told you.

Ten minutes later my hand hurt; it bleeding.

I spoke, real words. I sat up and watched the world get a little smaller and let me step back into it. I hugged my girlfriend. I called my dad. I moved back to Ohio. I started living.

TIA

I had a TIA (transient ischemic attack). A TIA is "stroke-like, lasts for 20-minutes up to two hours, and then goes away. It's like a warning. Your body says "Change something dude, or I'm gonna change you".

I can't say I was immediately transformed into a monk walking the diet line anointing those I met. I can say, however, that it opened my eyes and I started learning. Truly learning.

No longer was I interested in eating 10,000 Calories a day in an effort to be a professional bodybuilder. No longer was I going to avoid all cardiovascular activity in exchange for bicep curls. No longer was I going to use the offseason as an excuse.

The day I almost died set me in motion. Motion is the best cure.

I don't want to leave the world feeling like I did while I was staring at the ceiling, carrying bags of guilt to the afterlife. Health isn't secondary, it's priority, and death isn't distant, it's right around the corner.

"The day I almost died is the day I began living."

CHAPTER 22

Protein, Cherry Picking, And Meta-researchers Are Rockstars

It was well past midnight and I wasn't having a nightmare, I was getting a call about food.

I tapped "answer" and before the phone reached my ear, I could here my friend Dave shouting obscenities my way. I waited until he stopped talking, then waited some more.

"Say something asshole," Dave said.

I laughed as best as I could for just being rudely awakened. Dave chuckled too.

Dave is a professional soccer player and a cowboy scientist like me. He loves to try new things and make sure what he is doing is the right thing.

"Know anything about the China Study?," Dave asked.

"Yup … "

"Can you elaborate or do I have to pay you … prick?"

"Can't we talk at a more human hour, Dave ... wait, is this for a woman? Are you dating a Vegan?"

"First, don't ever lecture me about women. Second, it's not about a woman, my coach is trying to get the whole team to give up meat."

"Got it. So he's dating a Vegan."

Protein

Protein, like fat, is an essential nutrient. Meaning, we need to eat it to live. Protein broken down is called amino acids.

Arguably, there is about 23 different amino acids. Nine essential, the rest non-essential.

There are ketogenic amino's that can't be converted to sugar, and there are glycogenic aminos, such as glutamine, which can be converted to sugar. This is why alcoholics bridge their sugar addiction with glutamine.

As we mention in our vegetarian chapter, complete protein comes from animal sources. Not soy, greens or nuts. In the Paleo Solution, by Rob Wolff, he calls those "third world protein sources."

Since protein is essential to live, and you can't get complete sources from plants or beans or nuts; then why the fuss?

Humans, simply, won't admit when they're wrong. Or more importantly, when the other guy is right.

Bodybuilders, Vegans and Christians:

In my competitive bodybuilding days, I ate two grams of protein per pound of bodyweight everyday. At 200 lb., that's 400 gram a day. I almost swore off chicken forever.

Four-hundred-grams of protein a day is about 50-grams of protein per meal if I ingested eight meals/day ... which I did. Everyone in the gym did. It didn't feel quite right, but since all the big kids were doing it ...!

Thankfully, I learned much. Yes, physique athletes eat tons of protein and sometimes they look great, but that doesn't make it the right, or easy for that matter. This type of high-protein/low-fat diet, the one that is most widely prescribed to the nation, is just a delayed carbohydrate diet with a fad name.

Sleeper carbs

When we stop eating fat, our body looks for something to burn. If we're not eating carbohydrates and there's no glucose to burn, our body turns to protein for fuel.

Massive protein diets add to the "flexible" or "liable" amino acid pool. All that excess protein gets a trip to a confined swimming hole ready for use later. Since it's not required to repair muscle, all that available protein goes through a process called gluconeogenesis (converted to sugar).

This is how too much protein makes us fat. We absorb it all, just not as muscle. In fact, it's not even just the abundance of one macronutrient, it's the lack of another.

Vegans got a point

It's not often I get to celebrate our non-meat eating friends. But when I can, I want them to know I care and I appreciate all they do.

Those who refrain from eating meat because they wish not to hurt another living thing are incredible individuals who should be rewarded for their great sacrifice and honored for their diligence.

The ones who believe it's healthier to be an herbivore, while I may disagree, need still be respected for the discipline required and the lessons gained.

If you know anything about non-meat eaters, you know that they have to perform some nutritional gymnastics to ensure they do not become nutrient deficient. Their goal is to group certain food together in an effort to make complete proteins and efficient nutrient absorption.

This ability to constantly put together different dishes in the kitchen is something Paleo dieters would do well to copy. All too often we get comfortable with eating the exact same thing everyday. This is cool if we cover all nutrient bases, not so cool when you're missing something.

Switch your protein from eggs, turkey, fish, and beef often. Try different veggies at every meal. Add crazy spices and coconut, olive oil and various nuts while experimenting with ghee and the like. The goal is to dabble, not get bored.

Christian Health and protein recycling

The goal of a "protein rich diet" should be that of "enough protein." Quality protein at that; meat eggs, fish and chicken.

Through fasting, as mentioned elsewhere, we can take advantage of protein recycling, or Autophagy. Autophagy is like cleaning house on degraded protein reserves, and it only takes 17 hours of protein avoidance.

Combining bouts of autophagy with a high-fat diet and a low-carb diet, allows us to remain in ketosis. Ketosis prevents muscle breakdown. Meaning, we can get by on much much less protein than I or anyone in the industry could've imagined.

Basically, we combine ketosis, autophagy, fasting, and Paleo.

Dosage

It's a challenge to eat 400-grams of protein a day. Eighty grams or so, not so challenging.

First, makes sure you're not measuring the protein in anything other than meat. Again, nuts seeds and the like don't count as protein, they can count as calories. For now, just measure the protein in meat.

If you're cycling your meal times, you won't get the same amount of protein everyday and that's great. Don't think daily Calories or ratios, think weekly and even monthly

Overdose
Somewhere along the way, someone labeled diets containing 20-29% protein, high-protein diets. As you may have guessed, 30% and above is cleverly named, very-high-protein diets.

Namesakes were chosen due to the upper limit of protein humans are comfortably able to consume on a "regular" basis. Researchers reveals that protein Calorie consumption, amounting to 35-percent or more total Calories per day, can end in a condition known as "rabbit starvation."

When protein breaks down it creates nitrogen which is fine and necessary. However, when we eat more protein than what our kidneys and liver can filter we become toxic.

Quickly, excess nitrogen is converted to urea which then begins to hinder the body by saturating the blood stream until our internal filters can't get rid of it. This is why all those bodybuilders, and super high-protein dieters smell like ammonia.

For a time, I got nearly 50-percent of my Calories from protein. My head hurt, my joints ached and my skin looked like like plastic.

Eventually, enough was enough and I began to experiment. Now, I lean towards 30/50/20 (protein, fat, carbs) and 20/50/30 (protein, fat, carbs).

Take it from the guy who consumed over 400 grams of protein/day; there is too much of a good thing.

The China Study

In 2005, T. Colin Campbell, published "The China Study." A book dedicated to exposing meat for the horrors it causes.

Dr. Campbell was funded by Cornell University. He calls his 20-year study, "The most comprehensive study of nutrition ever conducted."

I bet The Weston A. Price foundation, and The Framingham Study have a thing or two to say about that.

Supposedly, Dr. Campbell was a meat advocate, and through trial and error discovered meat, somehow, was the cause of liver disease, cancer and war in the middle east. Well, maybe not that one, but the guy lays some pretty audacious claims. Claims, that are of course, backed up by his 20 years of research. Research funded by people with an agenda.

Unless you're willing to put the studies to the test, there is virtually no way to guarantee their findings.

The guys paying the grants are looking for specific feedback. If the scientists running the studies don't give them what they're looking for, they lose funding.

Denise Minger and Meta-researchers

Denise Minger from rawfoodsos.com, is a meta-researcher. You can find her extensive work against the China Study via her web address above.

Meta can mean "beyond" or "after." So, a meta-researcher is someone that goes in and researches the researchers. Meta-researchers today, usually paid for by competing companies, disprove about 85-percent of what we are originally sold as a nation.

Thankfully, we're all born meta-researchers like Denise. We have the power to put the tests to the test, and see what happens. I did. When I tested a meat-less diet, everything sucked.

As long as were are objective we will always find the truth amongst the lies.
At Denise's website, she has clear and concise proof of scientific cherry picking. Showing only the data that supports your theory, while hiding everything that doesn't.

Dr. Campbell had a an agenda that wasn't about finding the right answers, it was about finding the answers he wanted.

λ

The sun wasn't shining yet, but it was close and I was tired of calming Dave down.

"Can you talk to my coach?," Dave asked.

"If you'll let me go back to sleep, I'll think about it. But don't get your hopes up, Dave. This one is like religion or politics. Once someone is sold on not eating meat or that protein is a cardinal sin, even death won't make them repent."

CHAPTER 23

BD's

I could read those swollen eyes a mile away. Angie was about to explode.

Had she seen me? Yes, she had, I'm not The Predator ... yet.

Still, I could make up an excuse, I could act like I'm answering my phone that was on silent, or quickly walk over to someone, anyone in the immediate vicinity like it was some kind of pre-determined appointment.

"Josh, we need to talk," Angie said.

Too late.

Like a geyser scheduled to go off at the same time everyday, she erupted. It was about food at first, then her family, then work. It happened so frequently I became a professional at faking interest while mentally taking a vacation. I jumped back to the morning, when everything was grand and no one was complaining.

My day started, as it often does, without an alarm clock. My first stop was the gym, one of my favorite spots on the planet. And not because I love working hard, because I love how it feels when I'm done.

After that I usually head to a coffee shop for headphones and computer screens. I write and read email after email, most boring, some inspirational: One girl I'd been working with for a month or so had just got on the scale. It said she lost 15 lb. One man finally got a pull-up. Several people were looking for CrossFit advice. Awesome.

"Sorry to bother you, but I wanted to say thanks," a middle aged women interrupted my coffee/email/author time. I removed my headphones that were more effect than necessity.

"You see, I came to a seminar you held last year, I haven't started working out yet, but I took your food advice to heart. I have been mostly Paleo for a year. I've lost 30 lb. and my son has lost ten. Thank you, and please keep up what your doing, it's helping."

She turned and walked away.

"I really appreciate that," I managed before she was too far to hear.

I walked a little taller the reminder the day. I was fulfilled. Blessed.

But life is as tricky as driving in a snowstorm. It pushes you to the highest mountain, just to knock you off it. When you're charged and ready to attack the world, you smell like effort and confidence and daisies. It's an aroma "Battery Drainers" (BDs) can't deny, humans who live by feeding on the happiness of others.

Your success, their kryptonite
The most successful people in the world have one thing in common: They surround themselves with other successful people. We get that. Maybe the most profound realization to this story isn't who they surround themselves with, but who they don't.

You would never catch our world's lightest and brightest hanging out with negative Nancy all the time. The most successful people in the world aren't better at finding a group of supporters. They are better at killing vampires.

BDs are those kind people who enjoy martyrdom as long as there is someone around to see them being sacrificed. BDs have a universal cold relationship temperature and they are always looking to steal a little juice from the warm burden carriers with quickly rechargeable batteries. BD's are not necessarily bad people, they just do bad things.

Families friends and you

A very painful, and very necessary realization, is the fact that the nation is dying. Maybe that's obvious. Maybe the more painful, and more secretive realization, is that your friends family and even yourself are very much part of the problem, if you're not actively producing a solution.

Since you're here - reading - I choose to believe you want a change. A worldly, meaningful change.

Transference

First, know your enemy by knowing yourself.

A husband who doesn't want go paleo or do CrossFit may be your BD. Or maybe you've done a million diets over the years and he's sick of participating in your passing fancy of an eating program every two weeks. Give him time to come around and don't shovel thrusters and almonds down his throat. Even if he never wants to participate, but supports you, he's a good dude.

Making someone a BD because they don't agree or want what you do is communism.

Transference is when you toss your insecurity onto another because the burden of your change is to hard to carry. When defining your BD's that have souls, make sure you're not setting up franchises full of people you can be pissed at when you fail.

"You would never catch our world's lightest and brightest hanging out with negative Nancy all the time. The most successful people in the world aren't better at finding a group of supporters. They are better at killing vampires."

Ask the hard questions about why you haven't succeeded before now. Then, objectively spot the true vampires amidst the more sanguine of the lost who may do everything to support you, but who wish to be nothing like you.

Picasso:
Once you've spotted the source of your lost energy, remember, the more you look like a unique painting, the more you stand out to the copies.

Your projection of strength will reflect the weakness of others right back at them. Your excitement will become their vehicle driving indignation at every turn.

They see you as a better, and since they don't want to improve, they will just make you worse. Have you heard this before?

"Oh, just have a piece, it won't hurt."

"Can't you just miss this one workout, you're there all the time."

"Why do you want to be in better shape, who are your trying to impress? I love you just like you are."

These situations, and there are many more, left unchecked keep even the best of us down. The secret to becoming, and remaining, a Mona

Lisa in a room full of comic books is simple. Shut-up, and keep moving forward.

"Making someone a BD because they don't agree or want what you do is communism."

Until you're well prepared with intellect, and ready to withstand any and every attack, keep your newly found fountain of youth a secret from those who would try to squash it.

Market your lifestyle with your glow instead of your mouth. This is living faith, not preaching it. This makes converts not enemies.

Technology:
While most Battery Drainers are human, some slide well under the radar with no pulse at all.

Technology is a Facebook page that never sleeps. Xbox gamers from two continents over. A flat screen+DVR in every room so we never miss a movie moment.

Progress makes like easier and people soft. We forget that with every new technological advance comes the cost of discipline to use it.

Realize that there is "too far" when it comes to the tecky side of life. Most times you just gotta turn the TV off, and airplane mode the phone to hear that little voice shouting, "help" way back in your mind hoping you will one day have the discipline to listen.

"Market your lifestyle with your glow instead of your mouth. This is living faith, not preaching it. This makes converts not enemies."

Our success is often related to the level of discomfort we're willing to accept.

As I write this I am alone. I hate being alone. But I had a deadline to make with this book. A deadline that was self-imposed.

I scheduled a lonely, week long sabbatical to knock out my remaining chapters. I love writing, but I hate this. However, it's when we are the most uncomfortable that we are able to shine. When we pay the piper in the present, we are blessed in the future.

You
You know just as well as I do, that we are our own worst enemies.

For years we spend time defining ourselves by our activities, our passions, our friends. Then, when it comes time to change, we freak out.

After a lifetime of creating our image, we become defined by what we cannot give-up.

Radical changes produce radically different versions of ourselves. They may look nothing like the happy-go-lucky drinker, or all-night-partier. We become very different and different is exactly what we are looking for.

⚓

"Angie", I said after half listening to yet another story about her cat, boss, fat ass or something.

"I dig you when you're happy, and I do enjoy helping people through tough situations, but I can't live your life for you. And your life is bringing me down. It's bringing you down too. I can't tell you exactly what it is, but I think you know what to do and the stress of not doing it is driving you crazy. Angie ... you're on your own."

CHAPTER 24

WHY NOT FRUIT

Well, that went greeeeat, I thought after speaking in front of a women's empowerment gathering in southern Ohio.

Risky isn't quite the word for it. More like tightroping over a lion's den with a ribeye belt.

My job was to be honest. Tell thousands of women how to lose weight. That it actually takes effort. I told them to take responsibility for their own lives.

"You even pissed me off and I know you," my friend said backstage after I asked how I did.

My pre-speech pep-talk was all spartan battle formation. The lady with the secret service earpiece collected me from the VIP room and walked me down a dark hall full of black curtains and speaker wire. I imagined the guillotine waiting across the stage for the crappy performers, donuts and medals for the winners.

"Be brief and be bold," she said.

"Hey, isn't that from toastmasters?," I asked. She wasn't amused.

"Communicate your most valid points, motivate them, then get off the stage and let the next speaker go," she said.

Every backstage smells the same. Oil mixed with seat and roadie smoke. I watched the cancer lady and thought I should stand farther away from the edge than she did. After all, those cured of cancer always seemed to creep up on the edge of things, like life didn't scare them so much as the rest of us.

She spoke like Beethoven played. Her testimonial lulled the audience like a serenade for lovers only. The crowd leaned towards the stage, and so did I, when she talked about her husband standing beside her when she shaved her head, he having shaved his own hours before, Kleenex made millions, the audience applauded. How do you follow that?

A green stage light shined. That meant I was on. I looked back at the secret service stage director as if to say, "seriously." The blonde in all black smiled back as if to say, "screw you and your toastmasters."

During my seminars I see the madness well up in the faces of certain crowd goers who believe Paleo is a total sham. Either my charisma (doubtful), or ability to read this from the stage generally soothes most of the wayward souls. At least to the point where they may just brush me aside as another diet guy.

But I didn't have that kinda time. My usually hour seminar was trimmed to a lean 15-minutes, clock sitting just to my right in big blue digital letters. It was like trying to disarm an a-bomb and losing.

"Women want to feel good, and they want the truth," my friend said backstage moments ago. It's all I could think of staring into the dark. With warm lights shining on my head like a sun drenched day at the beach, I began. Fifteen minutes later, the coordinator of the event hustled me off stage.

Free, I could leave, out the back of course. But I stayed. I was curious like Alice in Wonderland. I wanted to find out what I could learn from 40-something, mostly overweight, hardworking females. Even though every one of them reminded me of my mom, the beautiful woman who raised me alone without her husband.

It reminded me of another time in my life, a few years prior, an all black live action comedy show in a part of town that was considered - you guessed it - black. I felt like I belonged until the actors on stage started making stereotypical jokes about black people. Funny ones that I didn't think I should laugh at. Jokes that I thought were secrets, skits that would be cancelled if the cast knew I was in the audience.

The longer theses women spoke, the more it reminded me of things I wasn't sure I was suppose to know.

I realized some very critical information that has stayed with me ever since. Information millions of women could use to change their entire lives in an instant.

If they cry they buy
To girls, crying is contagious.

When I was working with a diet company many years ago, their sales leader, a woman, said, "bring back all those painful memories from their past, remind them of why they're fat. When they cry they buy."

I left the company the next day. The orientation was more like guided manipulation. A blueprint for scamming fat women out of their money by making them feel bad about themselves. I'm all for honesty, but there's truth, and then there's feeling like I need to shower in acid.

Women have an emotional capacity that men will never know. This is a great source of their strength, but left uncontrolled, it becomes a weakness.

I'm not saying men don't have some of these same issues, but I'm saying that women let their emotions stop their progress. They tend to create situations where situations don't exist. They beat themselves up over everything. They carry failure like a handbag three years out of style.

Women are their own worst enemy, but once they get it, they're more focused than a million telescopes.

Women Together

I have found on more than one occasion that women, much more so than men, create more problems than they solve when they gather. Admittedly this is not gospel, but the adage usually holds true.

When men get together we are definitely bring our fair share of dysfunction. We usually drink or play games and avoid conversation about feelings. But on the rare occasion when we do talk about relationships, we almost berate one another for the stupid actions he's done. We never console each other, more like condemn.

Men ridicule idiocy, women excuse it.

If I was to recount any story to a group of guys, they would question me. They would only comment on me, the part of the story they were getting told. It's unfair to give comments to, or about, a person who isn't there to defend themselves. Guys know this, it's called talking behind people's backs and we hate it.

The table full of males would call shenanigans over everything stupid. And we rarely praise the good. After all, good is expected, why get applauded for doing the minimum.

Typically, women get together to form accountability tribes. Great idea. However, be aware that accountability quickly becomes group justification if even one weed is allowed to grow.

I stuck around to the end of the seminar to see if I'd be stoned. To my surprise, I was swarmed, blasted with questions about the simple and quick tips I gave; one being give up fruit. "Why not fruit?"

A Fruity Situation:

Removing the last sweet stronghold for sugar addicts is no different than closing down the crack house on the corner.

Sugar is as addictive as cocaine and instead of trying to find reasons, facts and falsehoods to keep snorting it, just step away from the lines on the table. After all, it is hard to see the truth when you're face down in a pile of white powder, or a bushel of apples for that matter.

Most of us grow up believing in the government provided food pyramid, now called Myplate. We accept it as gospel but argue with the tax man.

Fruit is usually a ripened ovary of a plant with seeds. It's generally not leafy or flowery like vegetables. Fruit grows virtually all over the world depending on climate and is a great source of vitamins and minerals and energy.

Fruit contains fiber which is why some people say they eat it … but that's a lie because vegetables have fiber without the sugar.

Actually, fruit contains two kinds of sugar. Glucose and Fructose. The ratio differs as does the vitamin and fiber content depending on the fruit.

Fructose makes you fat:
Fructose is a simple sugar, meaning it doesn't really get broken down to become adsorbed, it's shuttled right to where it needs to go. The difference of fructose and all other forms of sugar is it's desired location. Fructose needs to go straight to fat stores (energy reserves), that's why God gave it to us.

The liver is essentially the central hub of the metabolism. It processes sunlight, manufactures cholesterol, detoxifies, stores energy and gives it, produces bile and regulates hormones. It also deals with fructose.

Fructose, unlike other simple sugars, cannot reload the muscles with glycogen after exertion, it can either stock the liver with glycogen, which is generally full from all the other food we ingest, or it can add to fat stores.

Fructose is digested in the small intestine and transported to the liver by the portal vein. An enzymatic process beginning with fructokinase, a compound confined within the liver. The reason this compound is housed in the liver is because fruit is not meant to go to muscles or other locations. Fruit's first target is the liver.

More than likely liver glycogen is topped off like a recently filled gas tank. Your body realizes that your tank is full, so it "reserves" that precious energy for later occasions where it can be helpful. This is actually fruit's main role and always has been. Reserved energy is also called fat.

Fructose Alzheimer's, cancer, Parkinson's and more
While fructose adds to our fatty outsides it reeks havoc on our our insides through glycation, in fact it's almost one fourth more glycating than glucose.

AGE's-Advanced Gylcation End-Products are created by the carbohydrates we eat. Fructose is a simple carbohydrate. As you recall, glucose by itself creates a wealth of problems we face today such as diabetes, Alzheimer's, Parkinson's and more, fructose is no different.

The diabetic argument is, "fruit doesn't make your pancreas secrete insulin." While that is oddly correct to a degree, the argument for becomes the argument against.

Insulin released is a biologically beneficial process by which our body mops up the toxic sugary compounds in the blood. Since this doesn't happen with fructose as it does with glucose, fructose stays in the bloodstream longer.

Thyroid, H1Ac, Triglycerides:
Not only has fructose been shown to dramatically increase glycation, but it also impairs thyroid function in several studies, making fat metabolism much harder than it rightfully should be. That means even if you should be burning fat, you won't.

If you're still not sold; get tested.

One of the health markers we love to measure, and maybe the best at predicting you imminent mortality, is hemoglobin A1c, or the measure of glycation (sugar) on red blood cells over several months. We are looking for a number of 5.0, or less. Add this number to your triglyceride (hopefully under 150 mg/dl) measurement which always is high when fruit is ingested because much more fat is created than necessary, and you have an internal toxic warning system begging for relief.

This is no mistake, fruit is supposed to do this. That's how we survived many years ago. Our ability to become unhealthy, followed by our ability to become healthy is what has allowed the human race to last this long. It's called seasons.

Paleo Fruitiness:

What lines the produce aisles today isn't exactly what our ancestors were eating generations ago. We've played Frankenstein with our fruit in hopes of eradicating the rather bitter tastes leaving only the sweet. So called "natural candy" that actually is three times sweeter than sucrose.

The fact that we can roll to any Whole Foods Market and leave with a bushel of whatever just adds to the dysfunction. When it comes to our food, there is no such thing as "seasonal." Today, it's always summer time.

An amazing book you should read and read again is, Lights Out; Sleep Sugar Survival, by T.S. Wiley.

To summarize lights out;

Summertime was a time presented to us to stay up all day, party like rockstars, eat plentiful amounts of food and prepare for hibernation. Now we have only summer. Now we have no hibernation.

Fruit was given to us to help along natural biological process such as diabetes, high blood pressure, and weight gain. In other words, to prepare us for imminent starvation/hibernation. As the seasons changed so did we, we fasted often, feed off our own "reserves" and came out on the other side no worse for wear.

Fruit is a gift given to make us fat and unhealthy, temporarily.

Fruit is a gift meant to be used sparingly as a means for survival, not a daily delight.

But What about our tropical ancestors:

Weston A Price, a dentist who traveled the world to study cultural relationships between man and food, came back with numerous studies of tropical tribes and diets. When we look to Mr Price we find a few consist observations which clear up the questions surrounding our warm climate ancestors. Those ancestors who live in perpetual summer.

1. A tribesmen along the equator still wearing a loincloth and smoking a pipe doesn't get genetically modified fruit like you or I. They get fruit that is mostly tart and full of fiber much more akin to a vegetable.
2. Warm living clans men are also ultra active. A typical day for an aborigine burns three to four times the calories of an average American.
3. The fruit they eat would be the worst thing they ate all day. Tribesmen do not have other forms of sugar, or too much of it. Tribesmen do not have fake fat, they only have animal fat.
4. Tribesman do not have abundance. Remember from our fasting chapter. A calorie deficient of poor food choices can still aid humans in certain situations.

HFCS and Fruit Juices:
Before I move on a comparison should be made between a bushel of grapes and Welch's grape juice.

One of the above contains a more refined version, less the fiber. One of the above is specially manufactured to taste sweeter than its more natural counterparts. Can you guess which is which? Now, does it really matter?

No. There is no difference. Once it's in you, your body just thinks it all sugar anyway. Your body can't read labels and it doesn't care if you can.

HFCS
We need to constantly look around and make sure we are not part of the majority. The majority is full of people who wanting to be a part of something right or wrong, willing to follow whomsoever speaks the loudest.

Be a minority.

Today the majority has geared their rage towards the detrimental effects of High Fructose Corn Syrup, a sweetener used in pop, candies and anything else processed, shelved and meant to be preserved much longer than it rightfully should be. Things loosely defined as food

HFCS is not even made from fruit, it's made from grain. HFCS undergoes an enzymatic process that changes it's glucose to a very sweet fructose so that less of it can be used. Essentially, more bang for the buck.

As of late HFCS have been targeted as painful, and full of dismay. This could not be more true. However, once again, like just about everything else the majority gets right, they miss the point entirely.

HFCS are a "loss leader". It's role today is to draw your attention away from everything else that is doing the exact same thing. After we bore of HFCS, we will just produce a different target to rally against making us forget the prison surrounding us.

It's wrong to make a distinction between HFCS, sucrose, and "natural" fructose. One is not bad or worse.

Bad is bad.

What's a fruit lover to do:
Years ago you gave up Twinkie's. Last year you even started to believe the hype about corn grains and beans. Today you're asked to give up the only real source of sweets you have, your only dessert and now you're pissed. So was I.

Like any other point in life you may not be ready for this truth. You may need to review your current plan and make several other exclusions before arriving at fruit elimination. However, fruit consumption may be the biggest obstacle in your way to success.

We've all been there. We all had help getting to this addicted spot by media propaganda, government shenanigans and devilish commercials. I never said leaving the hype for what's right was easy for everyone. If it was, obesity would not be epidemic, children wouldn't be fat and my dad would be alive.

Everyday under the spell of society is cumulative. Everyday we make excuses is another day we could have made changes. Everyday we find a reason that it's too hard, we miss the reason that it's so important.

I urge you to leave your taste buds out of the argument and come to the realization that every good thing contained in fruit is presented with the toxic wrapping paper of fructose. Sure there is a reason, but in today's day and age we need little reason to put any more toxins into our body. And calling it nature's candy, labeling it natural doesn't make it healthy.

One of the biggest scams was claiming natural meant healthy. Hurricanes earthquakes and tornados are natural, and very unhealthy to many of us.

A fruitless 30 days is all you need to discharge the fruity dilemma from your life forever. I'm not saying you won't miss it, I'm saying what you gain from giving it up is monumental compared to the damage you do by defending it.

In Review:
Fructose makes you fat. That's its job.

Muscles, organs, and tissue are left wanting when Fructose is ingested. Fat cells, however, grow.

The thyroid gland is hampered greatly by fructose intake.

Fructose is over ¼ more glycating (rust producing) that regular sugar, and it doesn't release insulin to help it leave the blood stream faster.

Alzheimer's, Parkinson's and just about every other neurological disorder can be attributed to excessive fructose intake.

Triglycerides, a real measure of health unlike cholesterol, is increased whenever fructose is ingested. They have to be, fructose is converted to blood fat, which is what triglycerides are.

Fruit was available to our ancestors. Fruit to help quickly add layers of insulation for upcoming hibernation.

Fruit today is different than yesterday. Fruit yesterday was tart, and full of fiber. Fruit today is sweet and sugary.

Today hypocrites blame HFCS manufacturers for the nation's health woes, while they munch on an apple. They are one and the same.

H1Ac is one of the best measure for mortality we have. <5 mg/dl and you are sitting pretty. Eat fruit regularly and that will go up.

Drinking fruit juice is no different than Russian roulette. Play long enough and you never will play again.

Fructose, fruit and the like isn't one of those start eating less today kinda things. Its one of those alcoholic twelve step kind things where you do whatever you need to not have another taste starting right now.

Get your blood work done. Measure your body fat. Take before pictures.

At the very least give it an honest go for 30 days, and then, if you're still not sold, you can always add it right back in.

CHAPTER 25

THE ONLY SCALE IS FOR FOOD

My office door was closed.

My office door is never closed.

The door creaked as I entered, slowly, as if it was booby trapped with a bucket of water above it.

One of my female trainers was counseling an athlete who was blubbering, the kind of erratic sobbing that makes you think they'll suffocate if they keep it up.

My mind went wild. Did a family member die? Am I going to have to kill her husband who just hit her? Did she just put down the family pet and now has to go home and tell the kids?

Silently, I caught the eyes of my trainer and they said "go away, I will tell you later." I slinked out of my office fearing the worst. I prayed for the best.

Twenty minutes or so later, the tearful athlete gathered herself enough to bolt out a side door not letting me or anyone else see. "She only lost one pound," my trainer told me.

"Huh," I said.

"She only lost a pound, and she thought she would lose more."

"ARE YOU KIDDING ME. THAT SELFISH THING WAS BLUBBERING IN MY OFFICE FOR TWENTY MINUTES BECAUSE SHE STEPPED ON THE SCALE AND DIDN'T LIKE WHAT IT SAID."

"Calm down," my trainer said. "This is calm. I thought I had to go hunt down an abusive husband or bury sparky, not mop the floor from 'step on scale tears.'"

In the most political face she could maintain my female trainer said, "you just don't get women."

True statement. But do women even get women? For that matter, do they try to get men?

The only tombstones given in Sparta were for soldiers who died in battle and women who died giving birth. Thousands of years ago soldiers were selected for battle/suicides because of how strong their mothers were, not how strong the soldiers were. This is a woman's lineage.

The female athlete above spent 30 days on the challenge listed in this book. She ran the RXD blood work, got body fat measurements along with girth. She even worked up the courage to take before and after pics.

Over the challenge I saw the redness in her face dwindle as her blood pressure plummeted.

I saw her personality come out as her body changed.

She spoke first instead of waited to be spoken to. I saw that normally fully clothed physique start to show skin, then a little more, then more as she finally put on shorts for the first time in five years.

I saw her pull that self-proclaimed "big-ass" over the bar for the time in her life, then I saw her do it again.

She even blushed as a newbie asked her one day, "what do you do to get your butt?"

Then, on the 31st day, I watched her forget that and disregard all the amazing things she had achieved in 30 measly days. I watched her measure success by a single silly instruments instead of every tool in the box.

Step #1-Trade-Up
If you don't already own a food scale you're going to need one. No, I don't expect you to do this at restaurants or even for the rest of your life. But in the beginning, and on occasion, it will be nice to measure your Calories. Remember, Calories are just another name for drugs, and you would be pretty pissed, or dead, if your pharmacist didn't like to use his scale.

Once the food scale enters your home, throw away the one you stand on. Or at the very least have someone hide it, and at all costs avoid the temptation of weighing yourself anywhere else.

Step 2-Treadmills Suck, Quality is King
The majority of people working out today, in fitness centers all over America, jump on some sort of treadmill, elliptical, and call it quits.

Any trip to the cardio section of one of these mammoth health facilities will usually find the same thing: A whole mess of fat people staying fat on cardio machines reading magazines at a snail's pace.

Herd mentality is great if the herd is going in the right direction, but this a lot like going nowhere--slowly.

When it relates to food and exercise "Quality is King," and usually the herd has this all wrong.

But they're coming around.

The Cooper Institute released its new cardiovascular health finding in 2008. They rescinded their previous recommendation of long slow duration cardio, and promoted a more interval based method for a much shorter period of time.

CrossFit has been saying this forever.

Basically, working hard for a short period of time makes you better at everything; including working for a long time. However, working for a long time doesn't make you fit. It doesn't really make you better at anything.

The trade off is apparent: do more work in much less time and become fit - CrossFit. Spread work over a long time, become less fit - Not CrossFit.

Our fuel (food) is no different when it comes to quality. Meat is great, grass fed meat is better. Eggs are good, Omega 3 enriched organic eggs are better. Almost anything in a box is bad, almost anything hunted and killed is good. Get the picture?

The argument generally arises that eating healthy is more expensive. But have you ever done the math? Or more aptly put, do you want to pay for groceries now, or the Doctor later?

Grass fed meat, nuts seeds and organic greens can feed a hard working human for under $7/day, or $210/month, and more than likely less.

Herd sharing, buying in bulk and Co-ops can drastically reduce Paleo costs further. And if you're part of a valued CrossFit community, this is most likely already happening.

The average Starbuck's coffee costs $3.10. Eating for quality of life is like drinking two Starbuck a day.

Its never been about cost, it's about priorities. It's about excuses or lack thereof.

Step 3-Photographers and Architects
Photographers take pics, or give directions on how to take pictures. Do this as opposed to getting on the scale.

Enlist the help of a friend who can see you close to naked and snap at least three angles. Make sure they're clear and well lit. Pictures are taken in the same spot every time, same photographer, same clothes. Pictures show the outside you that's conforming to the changes happening on the inside.

Interestingly that is exactly how we change. The reason Buddha went into solitude and meditation for twenty-years was that he knew the value he could have to others if he was enlightened. He first worked on his inner self, the side effect was his outer blessing that changed the world. It may be sad to say, but fat on the outside still means somewhat deranged on the inside, and that always prevents the maximum amount of awesome we can offer others.

Take photos every two weeks for as long as it takes. No one else ever needs to see them, but if you really want fast paced results, someone should.

I spend many hours behind a computer screen observing pictures of athletes from all over the world. I am their coach, I hold them accountable.

Architects build scale models. Your picture is your model. Your "girth" measurement is your scale. Have the same friend measure your worst areas twice a month. Preferably waist, hips, thighs, chest, arms, quads. Compact muscle may add weight, but it won't take up more room. This is why the scale only helps scientists, it never helps the experiment.

I'm the scientist, you're the experiment. Act like it.

I could round this out with a tangible goal speech, explain how scientific methods are always observable, repeatable and empirical, but today, I don't care to.

Maybe somewhere down the line in this book we can talk about the goals you have for yourself projected in your mind like a cinematic masterpiece, but there are plenty of two bit charlatans selling "goals," and "don't kill yourself books," as it is. I'm not even sure if I believe goals are necessary.

Some say they need direction and firm goals provide that. But many of those same people spend so much time writing down actionable, definable, long term dreams, that they don't get anything done. I like to write down what I want to do today, spiritually, financially, whatever. Then, most importantly, I like to check it off.

The thing I do believe in is NOT being busy.

Busy is not productive and sometimes the most productive things are boring and hard to get motivated for. Once you find yourself completing your heart's passion first thing in the day, every day, then everything else just falls in line.

If you feel like you need direct goals, more power to you, but I believe our enteric nervous system has a subconscious goal for us. A sort of bodily set point. The enteric nervous system which has more nerves than the spine is located in our stomachs.

The visceral nerve connecting our gut and brain line the entire GI tract. We sense hunger, pain, emotion ... just about everything in our gut. Once it's not clouded with poison and allergens anymore, our body will go where it should, not necessarily towards some douchebag goal, or worse yet, some odd BMI measurement.

If your goals are simple; drink more water, eliminate poor food, eat nothing man-made while trading up for meats, nuts, seeds and greens there would be no need for anything else.

Daily changes amount to lifetimes of success.

Recognize every change and celebrate it. Don't pressure yourself into fitting into a pair of jeans you would have to cut 12 pounds of muscle off to slip over your thighs. Don't post a Victoria Secret skinny-fat model on your mirror and say, "that's the butt I want." That's her butt, and you can't have it, and hopefully, after reading this book, you want more than a saggy, flat posterior.

Conformity is the enemy of individuality and our media has sold conformity to such a degree that women try to fit where they don't belong, while men, not genetically gifted, find superstar workouts that don't make us superstars.

If our target is fitness, not image, health is the reward.

Trade that floor scale for a food scale, have a garage sale for your treadmill, take pics, get measured and workout hard and fast.

Don't spend time writing it all down or thinking it over, just call me in thirty days .. then we'll see if you still think you need a "goal."

CHAPTER 26

SUGAR AND KIDVERTISING

French researcher, Dr. Serge Ahmed, has been studying sugar and it's addictive connections for pretty much his entire life. The man is damn near 100-years-old. To his credit, he has maintained a sugar free lifestyle for almost his entire life.

His most interesting study to date, that I'm aware of anyway, is a study involving a whole mess of rats, some coke, and sugar.

Over his controlled study, Dr. Ahmed found what most of us already know to be true; Sugar is addictive.

What's interesting, is that when given the choice freely, rats chose the sugar long before the coke.

"When society finally discovers that refined sugar is just another white powder, along with pure cocaine, it will change its mind and attitude toward refined food addiction." - Dr Ahmed

Dr Ahmed goes on to explain that intense sweetness can intrigue even those of us addicted to substances other than sugar. Meaning, if you're already a coke head, and you eat enough sugar, you will crave more coke.

If that wasn't enough, the sugar was removed from each and every rat, and guess what? Withdraw. The rats exhibited classic withdrawal symptoms close to that of a morphine addict. They went into shock.

Lastly the rats were given the choice one more time. Sugar, even after all the pain it caused, or cocaine. The coke was left untouched, and the rats had their fill one last time.

We're the rats

I know we have beat the carbohydrate thing to death in previous chapters, and yes I know sugar is a carbohydrate and that if we are following the rest of this we are performing sugar prohibition anyway, but I wanted to show you just why it's so hard to overcome this white demon so you don't feel defeated when you feel like some back alley cupcake-junkie looking for your baker.

For sugar addicted adults all hope is not lost. Certain tactics below can help overcome the world's new white powder, for us, and maybe more importantly, our kids.

Kidvertising

The real victim of the war on sugar isn't me or you, it's the next generation growing up in this day and age when advertisers have all but perfected marketing strategies to keep kids craving.

Parents say;

"My kids won't eat that, I have to make them something else."
"Their friends would thinks 'its weird if they weren't allowed to eat ice cream."
"I refuse to deprive my child."

What they really mean;
"I don't want to change, my kids are my excuse."

"I feel weird not eating what everyone else does."

"I'm not depriving myself."

It's hard to give your kid a bottled water when other parents give their kids Gatorade, but think about how much better you would be today if someone had made those changes when you were young.

Personally, I found myself growing up in a sugary haze of a childhood obesity. What I would have given to have lived in one of those "mean" households. The one's who care enough to take cereal off the table and pop out of the fridge.

How to kick the white demon forever

1. Buy and stock lots of fatty Paleo foods. Bacon, nuts, coconut. These are the new treat.
2. Never, ever have sugar in the house.
3. Turn off the TV.
4. Reward kids and yourself with something other than food. Food should be a necessity not reward. Take them to an amusement park, let them get out of chores, throw a party, whatever doesn't have a taste.

Kids follow our examples not our beliefs. If we say sugar is bad, then slam it by doughnut dozens or serve it every morning, they'll grow up just like we did. Addicted, self-conscious and sluggish. On the other hand, if we put in the effort now we can win the battle without ever having to go to war.

Sugar abstinence starts with us, the adults, but it's for the good of generations to come, kids who never had a chance, staring at monitors with tailored Ads aimed at 7-year-old brains. It's criminal.

Big Soda, General Mills, all the guys with skin in the game in the form of syrup and addiction are praying we never wake up and that they can keep hypnotizing buyers from the cradle. Well this is your wake-up call. Don't do it for yourself, do it for them, the ones too young to fight for themselves. Stop the sugar gorge. End Kidvertising.

CHAPTER 27

BAPTIZED

I hated church when I was a kid

It's Sunday, for God's sake, can't He find another day to in the week to make us get up early, dress pretty and sit through fake school? And that lousy music they called hymns, seriously?

When I learned hypocrisy I hated it more. And not just because my mom's best defense was "because I said so," but because half the Christians, the ones I saw out in the world, did the exact opposite of what they were taught.

But Ryan made it better.

I met Ryan in fourth grade and he's been my best friend ever since. When I had sex for the first time with the dark-haired girl up the block, I told Ryan first. I was the best man in his wedding, there when his first kid was born, and if it wasn't for him all those years ago I may have given up church forever.

When we were kids he all but lived with me and my mom. Every Sunday she forced us both to church. We joked, pictured the cute teenage girls in the front pew naked, and passed the time drawing on bulletins.

While I was busy being offended, gaining a special sort of cynical I haven't since been able to shake, Ryan was paying attention. Ryan never payed attention. He was the kid who needed Ritalin every three-seconds, the guy who told the same story over and over again. What did he see that I didn't?

Years passed. Ryan lived the life, finding one perfect woman, respecting her, marrying her several years later; Christian as Christian gets. Meanwhile, I tagged everything that walked and ran as far as I could from the church I grew up in.

But I couldn't shake it. No matter how much I wanted Him to, Jesus wouldn't leave. Sometimes it was hard to see the signs and I felt alone. Others the message was clear; get your shit straight before it's too late.

When I needed him most, and more importantly when I was ready, Ryan was there.

"I want to get baptized," I said when I called.

A month later, with my mom and dad and friends and Ryan watching, I got dunked for God.

Since then I've gone a little easier on the Christians I used to hate. Hypocrisy, apparently, isn't always intentional and being a Christian is hard work. But Ryan never gave up on me. And unlike my mom all those years ago, he didn't shove Jesus down my throat. He lived it, as best he could, and I watched. When I was ready, and not a moment before, I took the plunge.

Chance are, you've already made the decision, that's why you're reading this book. But just because you've seen the light doesn't mean everyone else has.

Paleo is exciting. CrossFit is exhilarating. Living a fitness lifestyle is a drug without side effects. A drug we try to sell too often.

Just because your husband doesn't share your passion for burpees and bacon doesn't mean he doesn't love you. And that wife of yours can be supportive whether she wants to meet your CrossFit buddies or not. Remember that and don't be the asshole force feeding your lifestyle to everyone else.

Be excited. Be yourself. Be honest. When your friends, your wife or your husband are ready, they'll come around. Until then, be an example.

CHAPTER 28

THE THREE C'S

Janine was crying. She tried to hide it over the phone but the interruptions of silence, the catching of breath, I could hear tears.

She called me behind her husband's back, a middle aged mother of two with an ass that required two plane tickets (her words) and severe self-esteem issues more suited for a therapist.

The voice on the other end sounded like someone stranded on a dark country road, no lights and no help for miles.

Mark, Janine's husband, had started CrossFit a year ago. Mark loved the community immediately. Soon after Mark loved the results. By the time I received Janine's phone call he was four pant sizes in the negative and 40 lb. lighter. Janine on the other hand, never gave CrossFit a chance.

To make it worse, Mark found CrossFit through Diana, Janine's best friend. Diana started CrossFitting four months before Mark and miraculously lost her stubborn baby weight--even though her only kid was sixteen. Who knew baby weight held on for almost two decades?

By the time I spoke with Janine, she was psycho dreaming about shanking her husband in the shower. Oddly, this wasn't the first time I'd heard this sort of thing.

Janine had begun to hate Mark's excitement and Diana's energy. She never really told them this directly, of course, instead Janine expressed her resentment other ways.

It started with yelling at the kids when there was nothing to yell about. Quickly, it grew to talking about her husband's quirks behind his back. Everything he did, even when it had nothing to do with her, was a mistake she criticized. Diana wasn't off the hook either. Janine made sure that all their shared friends knew just how much of a home-wrecker Diana was. That you should lock your husband up whenever she's near.

"I get it Josh, you guys workout hard," Janine began. " It's not that I'm scared of the workout. I'm scared of the fact that you do it in such a large groups. I've quit every exercise program I've ever started, but I did them all alone, I've never failed in front of a group. Can you train me alone, and not tell Mark and Diana? I just couldn't take failing at what they love so much, but I can't take treating them poorly anymore either. Something has to change. And its me."

Janine wanted a chance with no strings attached. Enlightenment without suffering. If I agreed, I would have failed the test as a coach.

A coach designs a program that best accomplishes the task no matter the method. For Janine and others like her, she has tried just about every method in the book. Except the buddy system.

Janine desperately needed community, the one thing she was trying to avoid. Janine need accountability.

"I train athletes one-on-one all the time, but that's not what you need," I said in the most unwavering voice I could muster.

The next few seconds of silence felt like hours.

Three C's
Community not a crowd.

A crowd is a gathering of people. A globo-gym is a crowd. So is a store and a movie theatre. A community is a group that defines its success by the whole.

Communities become crowds when their members, who aren't really sold on this whole selfless attitude thing crave attention because they were messed up to begin with.

The best cure to a crowd is a CrossFit community. It will give you the world as long as your selfless enough to focus on making sure everyone gets their piece of heaven. When you think it's all about your own personal happiness, we will eat you alive.

The question is; does CrossFit deliver because you got your pull-up, or does CrossFit deliver because you got involved with a community far from the crowd that just happened to like pull-ups?

CrossFit is one of the most life changing communities on the planet. The land is littered with thousands of affiliates to chose from. The first life changing "C" is Community. A community you must have to hold you accountable while challenging you for more. The community found in CrossFit.

Consistency;
Ralph Waldo Emerson said, "Consistency is the hobgoblin of small minds." I believe he meant consistency as a synonym for stubbornness and failure to grow.

When we talk of consistency we mean the continued application of good habits that divert attention from addictions.

CrossFit preaches mechanics first--get it right before you do it fast. Most people hate starting out slow but this will save you a world of pain in the long run. In fact it's a natural state of life to learn to move before you can learn to move quickly.

The first life changing "C" is Community. A community you must have to hold you accountable while challenging you for more. The community found in CrossFit.

After most of the rudimentary mechanics are in the bag you gotta use them. Consistency follows mechanics. There is no reason to practice proper techniques if you don't employ them enough to work. No matter how good CrossFit is, it doesn't work if you don't do it.

Our bodies function best when we lay on the accelerator in short bursts, resting every few sunrises. Even those rest days should be full of actively. Learning new sports or games, playing with pets and kids.

Truth be told, I feel worse after a day off. This is all relative to how hard you push yourself and the quality of your food of course, but nine times out of ten I rest because I think I should, not because I want to.

Workout consistently, no less than 4 days a week, and if you can get away with more go for it. Remember, a workout can take less than 5 minutes if done right. Duration is deception, and consistent intensity = results.

Competition
The CrossFit Games are the world's premier test of fitness. There's nothing like it for proving fitness and there never will be.

The CrossFit community bore the Games through the competitive edge each and every community member cultivates. When you're standing in a room full of other fitness superstars, average folks, newbies and soccer moms, you just go harder than if you were alone.

Workout consistently, no less than 4 days a week, and if you can get away with more go for it. Remember, a workout can take less than 5 minutes if done right. Duration is deception, and consistent intensity = results.

Do you have to compete at The CrossFit Games to be fit? No. But you have to compete.

Competition begins inside us, even that guy who says he's doesn't have a competitive bone in his body, that's code for I hate losing so much I quit trying. I

The third "C" is competition. The sort of competition CrossFit is built on. Not you against the fittest man in the world, you against yourself. Make an honest look and measure yourself today, now beat that tomorrow.

Your Micro-environment

The three "C"s-Community, Consistency, and Competition- are more than a map to fitness. It works for everything; church, school, music. It's intrinsic. It's human.

Start by building or finding your community, then you can more easily become more consistent with the assistance of others, finally becoming intense enough for it all to work by way of competition. The pieces of the pie may not be equal but if you don't have the full circle, the filling will just spill out no matter the size of the hole.

The CrossFit community bore the Games through the competitive edge each and every community member cultivates. When you're standing in a room full of other fitness superstars, average folks, newbies and soccer moms, you just go harder than if you were alone.

I still talk to Janine, usually in the evening with the 5:30 CrossFit class she loves. She began three years ago.

To finally get her to commit, I grabbed a CrossFit veteran and asked if she would reach out to Janine. "Invite her to class, please." As expected, they became fast friends and Janine started coming on her own. I planted the seed of the community, the rest is history.

"It's the people that keep me coming back when the results don't seem like good enough motivation," she said.

CHAPTER 29

Supplements: The Sacred Six

"**We just want** to place our products on your shelves", he said urging a hand shake. "It will be my responsibility to stock inventory, all you have to do is sit back and watch the money come in. And of course, pay me my share."

The man in jeans and a Metallica shirt (I swear he bought it because that would make him fit in) was urging me to carry his products. Supplements he discovered a month ago. Now he was an expert.

After a product crash course by someone higher up the pyramid than him, he was smart enough to tell me what to do.

This cycle repeats itself frequently. "B" meets "C". "B" sells "C" on something "A" sold him on yesterday.

Essentially, all piano teachers need to do is stay one lesson ahead of the student.

"It's not that I have a disdain for capitalism or a distaste for profit", I said. "It's that I've done this for over 15 years and I've experimented with just about everything. Things I bought in cars from large, scary men, and things

I bought from GNC. You have no experience and no business pyramiding anything that has to do with health. Even if it worked, which it doesn't, I would refuse to buy it from you."

I bet he returned his Metallica shirt. Probably likes Blink 182, anyway.

Detours

There is, on average, 4,000 Calories created per day per American. If this seems like a lot it is. In fact, the food Americans waste due to improper handling, spoilage and poor management could likely feed all those hungry today.

Taco bell, Subway and the like are not the only ones to take advantage of this over consumption obsession. The supplement industry started small by claiming we need to eat frequent, small meals. They promised the more you eat the more you burn.

They forgot to mention that burning 10 extra Calories because you ate 100 is still bad math.

The supplement saboteurs regaled us with prescriptions of five to seven meals a day. We fell for it. Since we didn't want to cook all of those small meals, we started taking supplements.

Supplements

The supplement industry began years ago and has since created a few gems. Whey protein, fish oil, creatine - awesome. They've also done their best to confuse us and back false claims with bogus studies.

After my verbal tongue lashing my networking marketing friend said, "So what do you take"?

"I'm glad you asked ... "

Fish Oil

Fish oil is a great source of Omega 3 fatty acids. We quasi-described this in our saturated fat chapter. "Omega" just stands for the family of fat. The 3,6,9, describes where the first double-bond of carbon occurs on this poly-unsaturated fatty acid chain starting from the methyl end, as opposed to the carboxyl … stay with me.

Omega-3 fatty acids are essential, meaning our bodies can't make it. We must eat them to survive. EPA (Eicosapentanenoic Acid), DHA(Docosahexaenoic Acid) ALA Alpha-Linolenic Acid) are thought to be responsible for our super fantastic learning curve bringing us to the wonderfully intelligent folks we are today (well, as I write this anyway. Tomorrow they'll be the devil).

In prehistoric, or even pre-agricultural times, our diet was laden with this little anti-inflammatory cure.

Omega 6

There are other Omega's, but that is for Mary Enig to describe. I highly recommend her book, "Know your Fats." But for our purposes, we will just stay with the popular ones.

Linoleic, Gamma Linolenic, Dihomo-Gamma-Linolenic and Arachidonic acid make up the Omega 6 family and these are also essential.

We don't need to avoid all Omega-6 fats. It's that we need to stop eating so much of them.

In days past, humans consumed a ratio much closer to 1:1- n-3 to n-6. However, with worldwide consumption of refined oils and heavily processed food, our Omega-3/Omega-6 ratio becomes a staggering 1:20 (n-3 to n-6).

Six and sugar

Insulin rises when we eat carbs. Combine insulin with copious amounts of Omega 6 and inflammatory hormones called prostaglandins rise. Don't get me wrong, sometimes prostaglandins are great - healing after a workout, wound care and testosterone production. But with more money comes more taxes and when we cram too much bad fat in alongside too many carbs, well …

Too many carbs + too much weird fat + not enough quality fat =inflammation = death.

Even our source of Omega-3 are not what they used to be. Livestock fed grains produce unnaturally high ratios of n-3:n-6. Fish farmed instead of wild caught fish are nearly toxic and crops will soon be completely manufactured in a test-tube.

So what can we do? Will supplementation cure this?

No. There are no supplements that overcome bad. But they can enhance the good things we're already doing.

How to Fish Oil

Buy some then test it. The simplest way to test is to put the liquid from either (liquid or capsule) in the freezer for about two hours. If it freezes, discard it. If it's still liquid, you're cool. Again watch out for the guy claiming his brand is 95-percent more absorbable. In fact, that claim is always a lie. No one can tell you what you will absorb, because they have no clue what you're eating to either enhance, or hinder what they are selling you.

Dosage

There are a variety of formulas to follow and a laundry list of dosages. Some studies have shown 15 grams a day fights cancer. Others show more conservative numbers. A general rule I have witnessed success with is, 5 grams a day after a blood test. Three months later, after re-testing, check your C-reactive protein levels(measure of inflammation). If it is down, and you feel great. Awesome. If not you can play some more.

If you're one of those rebels unwilling to have a go in Dracula's office, you may simply divide your body weight by 10. Then multiply that number by .5 or 1 and there is your requirement. For example. I weigh 185/10=18.5x.5 = about 9 grams a day.

"No one can tell you what you will absorb, because they have no clue what you're eating to either enhance, or hinder what they are selling you."

Turn over your bottle and align that number with the amount of DHA, and EPA listed. If the bottle reads 1000 mg and only is comprised of 350 mg DHA, EPA put it back. We are looking for Omega-3 content. Insure that the pyramid guy isn't selling snake oil in place of fish oil. Hopefully, you can find a product that is almost entirely Omega 3(EPA, DHA) less the binders and fillers.

I like Purepharma a lot.

Notes
There are a couple things to think about with this supplement.

First, if you stay away from processed everything and only eat grass fed meat, you may not need it.

Second, this isn't Paleo so back off. This is about attaining a product that retards the action of living in such a challenging time. If you're not an athlete, sick, depressed, stressed then this may not be for you either.

Also, folks taking blood thinners like Warfarin and the like need to be careful, you can bleed out.

It's also worth noting that saturated fat increases the absorption of n-3 so keep up the coconut for yet another reason. The increasing Omega-3 absorption will also increase the demand for fat soluble vitamins A, D, E, K so be sure to keep Ghee on the shelves and Kale in the fridge.

You never know how bad you feel until you truly know what good is. Your dosage here, like the majority of this book is not so much gospel as example.

Hopefully, we awaken that little kids within you who loves to try new things and is willing to grasp hold of what works and pitch what doesn't. It's not about me giving you the exact dosage from one study one day in time. It's about me delivering pertinent information that I have tried and will guarantee with my life. Then, it's about you drawing your own conclusions after you try it.

Next, start by eliminating the items on the table that aid in that horrible western ratio we are trying to avoid:

Farmed fish
Grain feed animals
Trans fats
Hydrogenated oils
Dairy
Grains
Soy

Exchange them for these:

Grass fed animals.
Wild fish and game
Saturated fat from coconuts
Ghee

If you're still not on fishy pills, grassy beef, and fresh fish, then take a look below at the disorders Fish Oil is thought to improve or eliminate:

- ADHD
- Depression
- Inflammation
- Joint pain
- Alzheimer's
- Eye sight
- Arthritis
- Psoriasis
- Heart disease

There are more but I'm done gushing for now.

Vit-D

Vitamin-D shines in to brighten our day as necessary supplement number two. Oddly enough, Vit-D is a hormone, not a vitamin. I wonder what Vit-D sales would be if it was called hormone-D?

Adequate levels of Vit-D are linked to everything from social effectiveness disorder, to cancer. Vitamin D can;

- Improve cognitive ability
- Fight depression
- Ward off inflammation
- Heals wounds
- Fight heart disease
- Burns fat
- more

Obtaining this fat soluble hormone through exposure or diet is not something to take lightly. You can overdose, but Vitamin-D toxicity is nowhere near as prominent as Vitamin-D deficiency. Coincidentally, If "D" is deficient, its pretty much guaranteed calcium is too, along with A, E, and K. Not to mention a low HDL marker. Mood swings and dysfunctional sleep habits follow.

Sources

Vitamin-D is found in meat. Another high five for carnivores. Vitamin-D is obtained through sunlight and even tanning beds when sun is unavailable or inconvenient.

Since this devilish deficiency has been linked to breast cancer, ADHD and just about everything, big-pharma has begun to produce Ultra-D tabs that you can more or less OD on. For instance, when someone's Vitamin-D measures below normal, a doctor may choose to toss a couple huge tabs down their throat to quickly bring their levels back in check. It's just that important.

Dosage;

Some folks take to the streets and hang out in the sun for 10-20 minutes a day. Others slam a few thousands IU's every night. Just like fish oil, the best way to see how you stack up is to bleed.

A quick blood test shows deficiency in 9 out of 10 athletes I meet. As we included earlier, we are looking for an active Vitamin-D level of 50 ng/dl. A far cry from the recommended 25 ng/dl of today's society.

When viewing what "they" say is recommend ask yourself; "Is my game to thrive, or survive?"

If you're unwilling or can't afford to get pricked, you could start with an arbitrary experimental dosage of Vitamin D supplementation. No more than 3000 iu per day.

Zinc

Zinc is a mineral necessary for our survival like just about every other trace mineral we ingest. Zinc strengthens the immune system, aids in proper prostate functioning and ensures a healthy night's sleep.

Paleo followers who somehow believe working out is unnecessary, may not need for additional zinc in their diets. However, more athletically inclined humans may find adequate zinc difficult to ingest while diligently training.

"When viewing what "they" say is recommend ask yourself; "Is my game to thrive, or survive?""

I have experimented with hundreds of supplements over the last fifteen years. This chapter contains the few making the cut and zinc is one.

Dosage;

If you're an avid active human wanting a little more, add 20mg or so of zinc before bed. There is, however, a catch ...

Magnesium

The catch is don't add Zinc, unless you're willing to add Magnesium. They work synergistically to help you sleep, lower blood pressure, recover, smile and a few other very important human occurrences.

In fact, I once read an entire book devoted to the values of magnesium. I remember about a page of it.

Magnesium is spectacular for natural evening relaxing and testosterone boosting. It also improves circulation mitigates depression, reverses ADHD, improves sleep, and much more.

Dosage:
Up to 600 mg before bed with your Zinc should help you dream sweet nothing about wonderlands and desserts before you were Paleo.

Creatine:
Creatine has been around the workout world since I can remember. Creatine was all the rage when I was in high school. Guys would snort lines in the locker room and run around all wacked out acting like it was some sort of "roid rage."

Parents didn't help the matter. Societies increasing tendency to place blame instead of absorb it, left creatine holding the bag and research halting for quite sometime. Thankfully, times have changed. We know creatine won't kill, dehydrate or paralyze.

Creatine is a nutrient produced within our bodies. In fact it is non-essential meaning we can make it as well as attain it from meat and amino acids. Creatine acts as a cell volumizer along with an energy giver. It's essentially a source of ATP(adenosine tri-phosphate) which is what the mitochondria feed on.

By supplementing with creatine athletes may be able to take advantage of increased work capacity. While creatine is reserved in the body, exchanged and manufactured in the phospho-creatine system, it still can be sort of topped of or added too like a gas tank not quite empty.

During times of increased energy demand, almost specifically anaerobic demands, that extra creatine can add another five pounds to a lift, or a handful of successful reps. If you've been working out long enough, this is a big deal.

"Parents didn't help the matter. Societies increasing tendency to place blame instead of absorb it, left creatine holding the bag and research halting for quite sometime. Thankfully, times have changed. We know creatine won't kill, dehydrate or paralyze."

Creatine also helps to push water into cells (it doesn't dehydrate) making the quality of our very important tissue that much better. In fact, those supplementing with creatine often celebrate less joint pain.

Creatine also enhances ketogenic diets like the one we prescribe in this book. The mitochondria also thrives more efficiently off fat once in Ketosis along with the heart and kidneys. When you're carb starved, creatine helps fat to be burned as fuel as opposed to stored as insulation.

Side note.
I often get this question, so here it is:

Q.Josh, Ketosis definitely appears to work well for most, however as a 100m track sprinter, my training revolves around anaerobic bursts, and from what I have been informed, can only be fueled by readily available Glycogen stores fed by carbs. When I was in a ketogenic state, I couldn't finish a track session without cramping. Now I pre-load with sweet potato or pumpkin/yam and I am fine. So I guess I'm just asking, is this the best solution for sprinters?

A.Great question. CrossFitters and sprinters and the like work at peak levels of intensity. Glycogen will fuel these efforts. Carbohydrates make glycogen. Ketosis, however, does not prevent the muscle or liver from becoming engorged with glycogen, but it does help prevent muscle from being wasted by promoting fat from being burned for recovery.

Ketosis will lower triglycerides when your body breaks down fat in the blood. A byproduct of that breakdown is a glycerol molecule, otherwise known as glucose later to be turned to glycogen.

After you have officially shifted your metabolism to ketosis, your body will readily fill spent glycogen by breaking down fat.

Now, if you're working out once a day for basic health standards, then ketosis is fine for you. However, ketosis may not be the answer if you workout multiple times a day.

In that case, we add carbohydrates until we feel that performance has reached it's genetic potential. The key is to give the body what it needs, not too much.

If you're a workout fanatic, add carbohydrates slowly and mostly after training and at night.

Back to Creatine now.

Dosage:

After a 20 gram loading phase, lasting five days or so, you can maintain and benefit from 5-10 grams of creatine a day. Typically, I cycle creatine for eight weeks, followed by an 8 week recovery period where I abstain from it all together.

Whey Protein

Curds and whey isn't paleo, neither is going to the gym, using silverware or driving a car. But, like everything else, it it heals and doesn't hurt, go for it.

Whey protein is a predigested form of nutrients that seems to absorb faster than real food. After a workout whey can immediately repair damage by way of shuttling amino acids to stressed cells. Whey is also full of glycogenic amino's so any addition or "flexible" energy not needed for repair can be converted to glucose on the way to help stock the tanks of the muscles and liver, priming the pump for the next workout.

"Curds and whey isn't paleo, neither is going to the gym, using silver-ware or driving a car. "

Eating carbohydrates after a workout is fine. However, unless you're training again in less than 24-hours, it may be unnecessary. Especially if you're trying to burn fat.

I like Pure Selection.

Dosage;
For those of you who don't wanna go the whey route simply eat a post work-out real food meal of 30-40 grams of protein as soon as you feel able.

Lastly, forget all of the above if you're not willing to eliminate the other stuff holding you back. Otherwise, give the sacred six a try.

⅄

I saw my buddy the supplement salesman recently, he was wearing a tie and selling jewelry.

"Where's your Metallica T-shirt?," I asked.

Baffled, I told him when and where we had originally met.

"I gave that shit up a long time ago," he said "Wasn't making me any money."

Dieting, supplementation and fitness are as near and dear to me as pant-ing to an artist. I've spent nearly two decades studying, testing and practicing what I preach. I've painted my rite to give advice in blood.

What's Vitamin C's real name ? Have you actually trained for more than a week at the beginning of every year? If you weren't getting paid, would you still sell this shit?

Ask your supplement selling pyramid buddy that next time he tries to hock something your way. Am I saying you have to know everything about everything to help anyone, or that you even have to take it yourself? No. I'm saying there's people that know, and people that act like they do for money.

Choose wisely.

CHAPTER 30

VEGETARIANS

After seven years of marriage, he'd had it.

"No more brussels sprouts, damn it," he said.

It was weird, sitting in on a fight between husband and wife like a pastor trying to save a marriage, but what choice did I have? He was a CrossFitter, avid Paleo follower and life long meat eater. His wife, however, was a rookie vegetarian, against the eating of animals for nearly 18 months.

"Tell her it's unhealthy," he demanded in my office. "Tell her she's gonna die weak, skinny fat and … weak. Tell her steak is meant for eating."

Kim didn't fight Steven when he began CrossFit. But starting fitness is a lot different than giving up steak. Every chance he got Steve searched for evidence. A shred of misinformation here, a meager helping or quirky science there, all he wanted was beef and barbecues … and a wife to share it with.

"And it's "your job to convince her that eating meat is good for you," he said.

I felt a little hypocritical, living under a meat umbrella my whole life. What if these meatless wonders are on to something and I'm the stubborn one? What if being a vegetarian healthier than the alternative?

Only one way to find out; test it!

Paleo me:

FB-68
HDL-62
LDL-84
C-Reactive Protein-1
Triglycerides-110
Body Fat-10%

30 Days Later...

Vegan Me:

FB-86
HDL-41
LDL-98
C-Reactive Protein-2.2
Triglycerides-250
Body Fat-16%

Fasting Blood Glucose:
FBG is generally taken when you wake up in the morning. As a rule, we would would like our FBG to measure <80 mg/dl. Even though the ADA (American Diabetes Association) goes for <99. Remember we going for optimal, not survival.

FBG is just one link in a long chain, but it's a good one. Yes mine was still well under the ADA's recommendation, but look at the increase. That's a 20% hike. Coincidentally, whenever your FBG measures 83 mg/dl and above, you're three times more likely to become a future diabetic. Even though it's "recommended."

FBG anomaly:
There's always a catch. Some folks following a low carb Paleo diet score high on their FBG measurements.

Upon Carbohydrate restriction the body activates lipase which breaks down fat (this is a plus) and burns it off as esterified fatty acids - muscle fuel. Remaining glucose may be shuttled to the brain or red blood cells.

You will know this is happening if your FBG is higher than it should be and your triglycerides are ultra low. A Triglyceride has a glycerol molecule holding the fat together. When it gets broken down your FBG can go up because of the glycerol. To Back this up, the next test becomes imperative.

H1aC:
This measures the sugar/carbs you have ingested over the course of the last three months. Every 90 days your red blood cells recycle. But interestingly, these cells have been glycated - they had sugar attached to them. H1Ac measures carbohydrate intake over the last three months.

Look for a value of <5.3. Anything higher is demonstrating what I call sugar saturation, or advanced aging. After all, the reason we age is sugar: AGEs Advanced-Glycated-End products.

Cholesterol:
If you want the specifics of Cholesterol you won't get it here. There is no use copying what five minutes of google searching will bring to your table.

But simplified, cholesterol is the technical support line for the body, and it's suppose to be open 24-hours-a-day-7-days-a-week. When we decide to eat meat, greens, coconut and avoid grains, dairy and alcohol, the operator is ready for the call smiling and speaking clearly, answering on the first ring. When we decide to stray for far too long, the line gets crowded and we spend too much time on hold.

Naturally we produce around 2000 mg of cholesterol a day. We will never ingest anywhere close to that. Cholesterol is essential in every process of the body, especially healing. It's also very helpful if you're in the market for strength, fat burning and sanity.

Without cholesterol we couldn't rebuild.

It's a precursor to Vitamin D (which is a hormone), Progesterone, DHEA, Estrogen, and Testosterone. It's difficult to heal without estrogen, hard to burn fat without testosterone, and nearly impossible to be happy without all of them. In fact, the national reduction of cholesterol consumption, may have led to the boom in antidepressant medications. SSRI (selective serotonin reuptake inhibitors) sales are in the billions.

GB and Cholesterol:

Cholecystectomy, gallbladder surgery, is one of the most popular procedures performed in North America. And it's as unnecessary as sunglasses at night.

The Gallbladder is a pear-shaped organ which rests next to the liver. Its main purpose is to collect bile produced by the liver, which is later released to digest fat.

Bile is generally watery and causes no problems assuming the fat we eat is real. Real means the kind of fat we get from eating nuts, animals, and oils. But this isn't what we eat, now is it? The primary source of fat today is the hydrogenated and partially hydrogenated kind from rancid oils meant to prolong shelf life. Then, to make matters worse, we eat refined sugars and carbs from boxes and leave the green stuff in the ground.

Soon that watery bile becomes stagnant and full of rancid, indigestible floaties. It not only stagnates, but it clogs bile ducts with stones of calcium or cholesterol particles like some sort of beaver dam cutting off a water source to the towns below. Obviously this hurts, when things hurt we go to the doctor. And as any good physician would do, they fix the problem. I have no doubt that they would recommend a lifestyle change before the knife, if we listened, but we don't.

Just because you can live without a GB doesn't mean you want to. Taking bile salts, having issues absorbing vitamins A, D, E, K, sucks like an airport in a snowstorm.

And the gallbladder is just one of many important residents living in our stomachs. What about the immune system?

Over 80-percent of our body's total immune capability is in the intestines and stomach.

Serotonin supposedly plays a huge part in depression, psychosis and various bipolar disorders. And serotonin, whether it plays as big a role as we think it does or not, is still mainly produced in the gut.

But isn't there bad cholesterol?

HDL and LDL seem to be the only universal health terms. If HDL is high, and your LDL is low, you're great. Today those measures are a religion we live by. But HDL and LDL aren't even cholesterol; they're proteins that shuttle cholesterol to (HDL) or from (LDL) the liver.

It's true, stagnate LDL (low density lipids), and VLDL (very low density lipids) isn't good for the body. But why is it stagnant?

Carbohydrates are energy substrates. That means they're the first food the body wants to burn.

When that happens small particles of cholesterol congregate like punk-kids looking for trouble. Eventually they combine with the insulin carbohydrates create and they mesh with oxygen in the arteries. We call this plaque.

When you're good at burning carbs you're great at storing fat.

You may recall my LDL jumped up by about 15 percent and still remained <100 mg/dl while I was temporarily a vegetarian. My supposed good cholesterol took a dive of 25-percent. Should I be alarmed by this? No.

Just like FBG, HDL, and LDL are only two more links in a big chain. One odd link doesn't spell disaster just like one blown wheel doesn't total a car.

Triglycerides:
Paleo Josh's Triglycerides were 100 mg/dl while vegetarian Josh adopted a 30 day increase of 250 mg/dl. Now even the American Heart association recommends >150 mg/dl; citing anything over 200 mg/dl to increase our risk for heart disease by double.

About this time our chain of health looks strong and unbreakable, or weak and rusty.

Triglycerides (TAGS) are three kinds of fat. But what looks like bacon in the pan, smells like cake in the oven. TAGS are actually the measure of carbohydrates we eat by measuring the fat we're not burning.

The more Carbohydrates I ate, the more my Triglycerides went up. Add that to the rising cholesterol and you make the perfect average-normal-American.

C-Reactive Protein:
C-Reactive Protein is the measure of inflammation in the body.

Not all inflammation is bad; we actually need inflammatory hormones to survive, heal, become muscular and lean crime fighters in tights. But like any best friend, there is a time when enough is enough, and that healing becomes hurting.

The values we are generally looking for, regardless of every other biomarker, is <1.0. Paleo me is cool, vegetarian me is sore ... really sore.

For an alcoholic to feel hungover, he must stop drinking. Same goes for bad eating. To really know what great feels like, you have to give up bad. Only then will you truly have a comparison.

From Dr. Barry Sears to various other doctors across the country, all agree on one important thing: too much inflammation is bad

Body Fat:
A lot of humans today would be happy to walk around at 16-percent body fat. But speaking from someone who usually walks around at 10-12ish-percent, four whole percentage points in 30 days is like the difference of a sprinkle and a hurricane.

To make matters worse, the scale didn't change a bit, but I still got fatter when I stopped eating meat. And my clothes stopped fitting. Fat, after all, takes up more room than muscle does so even though the classic bathroom barometer of health didn't budge, my sides grew handles. And that's not all ...

Other Stuff That sucked while I was a vegetarian:
I bought new Clothes.

On the surface many of us would jump at the mid-life wardrobe call. But this curtain wasn't a fun intermission. This was a shrinking chest and shoulders - basically what makes a man look like a man was going away, while my waist was growing. Think hourglass, think girl.

All this even though I stayed away from estrogen producing compounds such as soy and the like. I simply wasn't stimulating enough testosterone.

Pissed off:
I was angry ... constantly.

Whiney:
I complained ... a lot.

Have you ever heard this?, "Now, I'm not trying to complain," or "I know this sounds like whining, but."

When I was a vegetarian I had a problem with everything God created.

And the crazy thing is, like most people living this way, I could see myself doing it and couldn't stop. I learned just how overwhelming our hormones can really be when spend every hour punching them in the face.

Ravenous Hunger:
The master hormone in our bodies lies within our fat cells; Leptin. It tells us when we're hungry if it's working right, if we're living right. To make it shut-u we fill its mouth with fat, to make it scream for more two-seconds after we've cleaned our plates, we can just keep eating carbs.

That's why sushi is like eating air and exactly why we stop for a steak on the way home from the Hibachi.

Vegetarians have limited access to protein. But fat should be nearly un-limited, right?

The Paleo me is about 60/20/20-fat/pro/carb. The vegetarian me suffered here. It seems meat protein played a nice role in digestion. The human digestive system has nearly 500 steps and the saturated fat from meat plays a significant role in that. Taking it out forced me to reduce fat which made me more hungry, which made me eat more Calories from carbohydrates.

The vegetarian me was 40/20/40-fat/pro/carb. I tried extra hard to keep my protein up but carbs jumped like they were on a trampoline. And since I was still doing my best to avoid allergens like grains, soy, and legumes, I was eating tons of greens.

The knife and fork are tools not friends:
I used to believe we needed to eat every two hours to stimulate our metabolism. I was wrong.

Eating every two hours is like tossing gas on a fire. Yes it flares up, but it's only burning the gas off. While we're constantly playing catch-up and burning that last meal, the body never has a chance to get ahead and tap into our endless fat reserves for fuel.

Eat less meals a day and release less insulin. Since insulin's basic function is energy storage (fat saving) then we become better at energy expenditure (fat burning).

In the end:
I tried. I didn't like being a vegetarian. If you do, good for you. I greatly respect your diligence and admire your convictions. But to me, being a vegetarian is just surviving, eating meat is thriving.

CHAPTER 31

DIETS DON'T FAIL BECAUSE OF DONUTS

I've been there, late at night, beneath the street lights and pale stars. Truck windows fogged, Kurt Cobain singing on the radio, Whooper in one hand, fries in the other, too disappointed to go home and face my brother.

He knew I was dieting and eating dinner from a sack wasn't exactly on the plan. So I parked three blocks away, ate like a addict and thought about hiding forever.

The problem was the plan.

"Failure, at least for me, smells like grilled beef, onions and mustard."

Back then diets were temporary. Something for a stage or a vacation, something I never planned on sticking too.

I learned the hard way that diets don't fail because of donuts, diets fail because we believe they'll end.

Eating healthy, living a better lifestyle, dieting; call it whatever the hell you want, is a lifelong commitment, not a quick fix.

After my second whooper went down with a side of disappointment, I drove home slowly thinking about explaining myself. What the hell is wrong with me, I thought, I'm not a cheating husband, I'm barely an adult eating Burger King. Failure, at least for me, smells like grilled beef, onions and mustard.

My brother never said a word. He didn't even notice. That made it worse.

That night I made a promise. No more quick fixes. No more getting ready for vacation. No more offseason.

That was a decade ago.

I can't say I've been perfect every day since, but I can say making Paleo a lifestyle was the simplest and most profound decision I've made. Nothing changed, but somehow, everything did.

CHAPTER 32

JUST TELL ME WHAT TO DO ALREADY

1. Go shopping

Everyone loves to buy things, that's why it's called retail therapy. Start your Paleo extravaganza far from the food isle. More like the stationary isle.

You need a journal. Almost all successful people journal something daily. Either feelings, pet peeves, future ideas, whatever. Not only will you be thankful for this daily analysis, but it may be able to help your friends will who undoubtedly want what you have.

While you're there, get a calendar to mark your start date. I say start date because there is no end to healthy. If you're looking at this as just another "fad" you are in for a rude awakening. Paleo living will change you and those around you more than you think. Simply tag your start date so you can periodically look at how long you have been going. Give it 30 days, then review, then give it another 30. It will be easier than you think. You will succeed.

2. CrossFit

Your community will keep you going when all you want to do is stop. Check out www.crossfit.com and map.crossfit.com to find an affiliate near you.

CrossFit is built for every body type and level of fitness there is. CrossFit is the actively we need and the accountability we can't live without.

Check my daily blog practicecrossfit.com, and joshbunch.com to find more paleo info, testimonials and articles dedicated to improving our lives and the lives of others.

3. Measure and Track
You need before pictures. Just do it.

I also urge you to get before markers;

- Waist
- Hips
- Thigh
- Body-fat
- Weight
- Blood Pressure
- Triglyceride
- HDL
- LDL
- Fasting Blood Glucose
- H1ac
- C-reactive protein
- Vitamin D

4. For the next thirty days, stop eating everything that is not; meats, nuts, seeds, vegetables, coconut.
You'll have withdrawal, it will pass and you will feel great.

5. Exchange carbohydrate for fat calories
Fat makes you feel full, carbs make you stop burning fat. Remove most carbs and until you start burning fat.

6. Eat coconut

We already have a straight-up coconut celebration chapter but if you have yet to start including it in just about every meal do so now. Coconut is a huge part of step five and makes dieting drastically simpler. I would play with the dosage, but a few tablespoons a day is a great start.

7. Eat meat

I'm not trying to pick on vegetarians, but if your protein source wasn't alive and at some point, then it really isn't protein. Every single meal from now on has meat.

8. Stop justifying

You may hit snag or two somewhere down the road. Don't let these blessings slip by without figuring out why they happened, and then ensuring they don't happen again. If we justify our bad behavior it continues. If we study it, we can discover the reason we fell off the path to begin with.

9. Don't eat fruit

It's sugar … stop it, seriously!

10. Sleep … a lot

I'm not the sleep guy, I'm the food good. If you want the 500 page reason why read "Lights Out, Sleep Sugar Survival." If you want the readers digest version, Sleep makes everything better, and we don't sleep near enough. Try for eight hours or more every night.

11. Stop eating breakfast

Breakfast is only the most important meal of the day to those people who sell it.

12. Fast

Not eating breakfast achieves most of our fasting benefits. If you consumed your last meal at 7 pm, then skipped breakfast eating your first meal at 12 pm the next day, you just fasted 17 hours.

My meal template looks like this;

- Protein 20-50 grams/meal of
    Beef
    Fish
    eggs
    chicken
    pork
    turkey
- Fat 60-150 grams/meal of
    Coconut
    ghee
    nuts
    olives
    seeds
    avocado
- Carbohydrates
    Spaghetti Squash
    Zucchini
    Green beans
    Asparagus
    Spinach
    Kale

For me, this simple template is a lifesaver. In a world where we worry about everything, not worrying about my next meal is a huge relief.

For some of you, this is too simple. You can easily Google Paleo foods and find ideas that will fit our guidelines. The only disadvantage is the more en-vogue Paleo is becoming, the more loose the guidelines. It's not easy, but it's simple. It's worth it. You'll be happy you did it.

CHAPTER 33

THANKS RICK

For a sixth-grader Rick was a giant, all arms and blonde hair, as big as the teachers and twice as big as me, the pudgiest kid in the fourth grade.

Before recess I prayed for rain. I could stay with my class that way, playing Sorry and drawing. Otherwise it was the Apocalypse, full of silver slides, monkey bars and Rick, the kid who taught me what a bully was.

If me and the rest of the fatties were lucky, the teachers on duty paid attention and Rick kept his distance. But most of the time something more important than a few missing fat kids got their attention, and Rick and his buddies made us man up on a brick wall while they hurled red, rubber balls and insults for 15-minutes straight.

And Rick was right.

I was fat. I did have boy boobs. I did weigh more than half the teachers. I couldn't run around the block, do a push-up or pull-up, or find clothes that fit. He was a prick and I wanted to curb that smile off his face forever, but he was right.

Like it or not, bullies like Rick are important. Motivating.

Because of Rick I began to dream of a time when I could run. When I could pull-up. When I was strong enough to fight back.

His taunts, as heartbreaking as they may have felt back then, were exactly what I needed. A spark lighting an eternal fire that would only grow with time.

Eventually, I got into sports and by the time I got to high school Rick was gone. That's really the only thing I regret. Part of my dream was meeting Rick on the monkey bars, little red dodgeball in hand, and saying "thank you." Thank you for making me hate unhealthy. Thank you for motivating me. Then punching him in the balls.

Who's your Rick?

Maybe your Rick is your fat father or your sick mom. Maybe it's the crippling idea of a nursing home or a wheelchair. Maybe you want to be an example for your kids.

The point is, I was fat when I was a kid and I overcame it. Then I found bodybuilding and got fat in a whole new way. But I never forgot Rick's lesson: no matter how far gone you think you are, no matter the names and the heartbreak, you're always strong enough to make a choice. Today, and for the last time, choose better.

Thanks Rick.

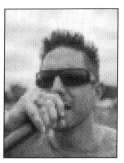

Since he was 18-years-old, Bunch has been all about fitness.

It started with personal training and nutrition. Then CrossFit happened. He hasn't looked back since.

Josh Bunch

Bunch is a CrossFit purist, a zealot for the fitness program he's seen help millions. By day he writes, plays with his dogs and writes some more. By night he coaches CrossFit and does fitness.

To contact email: practicecrossfit@gmail.com, search practicecrossfit.com joshbunch.com

Made in the USA
Middletown, DE
27 January 2018